Introduction

The Nervous System Treated Naturally is part of a series which goes through the different body systems, covering all the main common problems that we as humans may have to deal with in our lives. As time prods us along and we start getting old and don't feel so immortal anymore, we will all get into trouble at some time and for the unlucky ones it could be serious. A lot of us have been failed by modern medicine especially through the system and the costs, along with hospitals always being fill, with long waiting times. This series is designed to empower you, educate you, help you prevent conditions getting worse, and give you the knowledge you need to know and hopefully make you able to have a good understanding of your condition, when you need to see your doctor. In this book I give to you all the Herbal and Homoeopathic remedies to the conditions you see in the first part of the index, and we have a good look at all the really hard ones such as Anxiety, Depression, Chronic Fatigue and how to fix damaged nerves especially after Strokes along with the conditions mentioned in the index, you have to take the best from both worlds. Next we move on to the diet you need to look at for this system especially for certain diseases, adding also the Superfoods for that system, and nutritional supplements that may also help you. Next you will come to the main herbal which will give you a very in depth write up about the herbs along with Precautions, Contraindications and the usual dosages. Following that comes The Introduction to Herbal Medicine followed by Understanding Homoeopathy. There is more to medicine then just taking drugs, with common sense being the best medicine there is. When your body tells you there is something wrong pay attention and don't let it get worse. Then there are others like me who suffered from an Industrial Accident and still suffer decades later, and only God knows how many suffered road accidents. But that's life and the reality is you have to pick up the pieces and carry on. I hope these books make your life easier.

Mark Gilberd

Medical Herbalist, Homoeopath and Iridologist

Cover Picture supplied by Monika Grabkowska of **Unsplash**

Chamomile is one of our main remedies used in the Nervous System

The Nervous System

Effects of Aging on the Nervous System

The Nervous System
Effects of Aging on the Nervous System
The Brain

Your Short term memory and the ability to learn new material can be affected relatively early may be starting around 55 years and of course depending on how well you have looked after your brain and how much abuse it has had. Use it or lose it can sum up a lot of the problems at this stage so keep this in mind and frequently review the information you want to keep. At about age 70 verbal, vocabulary and stringing words together may begin to decline though intellectual performance and the ability to process information is usually maintained until about age 80 but again it's a case of use it or lose it in other words the info used recently or daily will have fast recall while something used 30 years ago may take time to put together again. Cells only have a certain time of life and as they expire the system will slow. The brains biggest enemies are depression, stroke, and degenerative brain disorders such as Alzheimer disease, Parkinson's and Dementia. Aging decreases the blood supply to the brain in the latter years by about 20% but this figure will vary especially in those with hardening and deposits in the arteries and the health of the heart. With less blood supply there is less oxygen which is why I always push Co Enzyme Q10 supplements but more importantly always carry them around with you for emergency situations. Take a seat, take a pill then start thinking what the hell am I to do.

Other Parts of the Body

As we age the Spinal cord can be affected from the wear and tear of life as the bones become hard and brittle and the disks loose there cushioning effect. Sometimes the bones overgrow causing Scoliosis or other nasty conditions that all have a chance of crushing or pinching a nerve which can lead to pain. Decreased sensation and loss of power. Peripheral nerves may conduct impulses more slowly causing decreased sensation, slower reflexes and the loss of smoothness and coordination in movements as the insulation layers around the nerves break down with Diabetes being a good example of a disease that accelerates this condition. Damage to the nervous system takes longer to repair or sometimes does not at all so care must be taken to avoid injuries.

Insomnia

Insomnia is a common sleep disorder which can be described as the Inability to sleep or to sleep for long lengths of time, or interrupted sleep. In other words persistent problems falling and staying asleep which has been happening over a long period of time. Most cases of insomnia are related to poor sleeping habits, depression, anxiety, being a worrier, lack of exercise and as in a lot of the aged a chronic illness that stops you from ever really getting comfortable which is a common problem of the aged. Another example is prostrate problems causing some to head to the toilet 3 to 4 times a night. Insomnia is not a disease in its self but can be a symptom of other diseases. Symptoms may be depression, anxiety, stress or difficulty falling or staying asleep and not feeling well rested or unrefreshed in the morning, can't sleep despite being tired, waking up frequently during the night, can't get back to sleep when awakened, waking up too early in the morning, daytime drowsiness, fatigue, or irritability, difficulty concentrating during the day and relying on sleeping pills or alcohol to fall asleep. Then there are problems that those have living next to a railway line, motorway or airport. Treatment for insomnia consists of improving sleeping habits and identifying and treating underlying causes such as room temperature, bad mattress or pillow etc try to make a nice environment for sleeping. Make a list and note down what you think are the causes that relate to you.

Herbal Treatment - Sometimes something really simple such as a warm bath with herbs such as Chamomile, Lime Blossoms and Valerian or essential oils (in small doses) like lavender, then off to bed can do the trick. Over the years I found the best way to go was to combine the powders of Valerian, Hops and Passion Flower into a large capsule and give this. Now you have to individualize this small dose to the patient so for example a patient suffering from anxiety and who is a natural worrier we would start them with a Calcium and Magnesium tablet earlier in the evening as worriers are always making the nerves do overtime and burning up calcium and magnesium and then give one capsule of the herbs. About an hour before bed give another capsule. If they want another capsule before sleep they can because in reality our capsule is a very low dose and if they wake up in the middle of the night they can take another. This is a example of going with the flow instead of the sledge hammer approach that you could buy in a herbal formula at any chemist. Each capsule has about 250mg of each of the herb and if taken this way for example you would only be getting 1000mg of Valerian where as in a chemist you would start at 1000 to 3000mg. The idea is to slowly move the body to sleep. The second herb we are using is Hops which is the main ingredient in beer and we all know in the aged that beer puts you to sleep fast even sitting up. Passion Flower the last herb not only has similar actions to the other herbs but is also a pain killer. Below are more sleep formulas.

Mediherbs Formula
Valerian
Passiflora
Skullcap
Capsicum
Weis says Passiflora is the best herb for intransigent insomnia - take 2mls before bed in water.

Powell -Associated with nervous and mental upset
Equal parts of
Hops
Passiflora
Skullcap
Valerian

Hoffmann
Equal parts of
Passiflora
Valerian
Take as tea before going to bed

Hewlett Parsons - due to pain or spasm, sedative, antispasmodic
Primrose 60g
Wood betony 30g
Simmer in 12oo mls of water. Take 50mls every 3 to 4 hours

Mittens' Formula
Passiflora 2 parts
Hops 1
Wild lettuce 1
Lime flowers 2
Take as a infusion, drink less tea and coffee and no heavy meals before bed

Powells general purpose nervine formula
Rauwolfia
Scullcap
Mistletoe
Sumbul

Hops
Humulus lupulus
Actions - Sedative, hypnotic, bitter, antiseptic, visceral antispasmodic, astringent, nervine.
Famed for its tonic and nervine properties, pain reliever, sleep inducer, antiseptic, tension that leads to restlessness, headache, indigestion, mucous colitis. Good for when digestive problems are caused by worry or nerves. One of the main remedies for IBS. Acts on the central nervous system and calms and eases anxiety. **Digestive System** – Nervous digestive conditions with insufficient secretions and over excitability of the nervous system. Visceral smooth muscle tensions affecting digestive and bowel functions, mucous colitis, spastic constipation, nervous dyspepsia, mucous colitis with Chamomile. Reduced stomach acidity, check fermentation. **Nervous System** – Sedative to encourage restful sleep, insomnia due to worry or nervous debility with Valerian, reduces symptoms of nervous

tension, nerve pains, excitability and hysteria with Valerian. **Doses** - Tincture 1 to 4mls 3 times daily, 1 teaspoon of dried flowers in tea 3 times a day or just before bed. **Caution** - Do not use in depression.

The Different Nerve Pains

Here we cover the different types of nerve pains and end with Shingles which at its worst has the whole lot at once, but is a good example of how a disease travels along the nerves and the serious damage it can do along with the speed it can do it.

Neuralgia

Neuralgia means pain of the nerves or severe pain along the course of a nerve. There are various causes including pressure on nerve trunks, faulty nerve nutrition, and an accumulation of toxins in the blood, inflammation of a nerve or nerve sheath or irritation of a nerve. It is aggravated by debility, anaemia and a rundown state of health. There may be local pain on the skin or right along a nerve, usually brought about by stress poor diet, lack of rest or infection. Causes can be aging along with chronic diseases such as diabetes or an infection such as shingles. Another nasty is Trigeminal neuralgia which is associated with pain from the trigeminal nerve which travels from the brain and branches to different parts of the face. Trigeminal neuralgia causes severe, recurrent pain in the face, usually on one side. It's most common in people who are older than 50 years. Have a look at the beginning of the Homoeopathy section to see what pains it can cause. Treatment for the pain of neuralgia depends on the cause and area of the body. **Herbal Treatment** - Focus on pain and cause. Infections must have fast and professional treatment such as blood tests to find the cause of the infection so as to relieve the swelling or other serious effects such as in Shingles for example damage to the eye nerves, always remember once a infection takes hold they can move fast. In chronic diseases such as Diabetes the damage is slowly but surely. In lots of nerve pain the problem can be caused by pressure on the nerve maybe from swelling, a tumour crushing the nerve or spinal disk or bone overgrowth. Here we will concentrate on Passion Flower which is a good pain killer mentioned before in shingles and we have the herb write up below. Again Chamomile is a good one to add as it is easy to find and has a good antispasmodic action as well as being loaded with Magnesium and Calcium. Add other herbs when you know what the cause of the trouble is. Following Pasion Flower are three professional formulas with Jamaican Dogwood and Devils Claw being another good pain killer.

Passion Flower

Actions - Sedative, antispasmodic, anodyne, relaxant, epilepsy, shingles, asthma, hypotensive.

A good herb for insomnia and a very effective herb for nerve pains especially in conditions like shingles. This herbs focus is more on restlessness and irritability, hysteria and anxiety and is soothing to the mentally worried and overworked it acts on nervousness especially due to unrest, agitation, worry, exhaustion and cerebral excitement. Used in the treatment of convulsions, epilepsy, tremors, hypertension, nervous breakdowns, migraines and neuralgias.

Doses - Tincture 1 to 4mls 3 times daily, 1 teaspoon of dried herb in tea 3 times daily.

Ligard and Halls Formula
Skullcap
Passiflora
Jamica dogwood
Gelsemium

For Teeth use Clove Oil. Ask at a Chemist, it's usually kept behind the counter.

Hoffmanns Formula
Ginseng Capsules
Hops
Jamaican dogwood
Passiflora
Pulsatilla
St John's Wort
Valerian

Oats

Mediherbs Formula
1. St John's Wort, sckull cap, damiana, Vervain.
2. Guaiiacum, celery seed, feverfew, birch, willowbark , devils claw.

Sciatica

The sciatic nerves branches from your lower back through your hips and buttocks and down each leg. Sciatica refers to pain that radiates along this nerve. Scatica occurs when the sciatic nerve becomes pinched usually by a herniated disk in your spine or by an overgrowth of bone on your vertebrae which is usually the cause when you get older or a impact accident in the area. Alternating heat and ice therapy can provide immediate relief of sciatic nerve pain. Ice can help reduce inflammation while heat encourages blood flow to the painful area which speeds healing. To a certain degree we have made a mechanical pump, cold contracts while heat expands so if you keep using hot and cold treatment you are constantly renewing the blood supply which brings in new nutrients and hopefully more of the formula you are trying to get to the area. Heat and ice may also help ease painful muscle spasms that often accompany sciatica. If symptoms do not go away you will need an x-ray and further investigations to rule out the nerve being compressed by bone or something else. **Herbal Treatment** - Here we will concentrate on pain relief and the antispasmodic herbs also look at St John's Wort in Neuritis and use this herb if the symptoms match. Black Cohosh will be our main herb here with the write up below. This herb is a anodyne which means pain killer and also a antispasmodic and with the action of vasodilator would improve the blood supply to the damaged area working well with the hot and cold treatment. Black Cohoshes Alterative action which means it is a blood cleanser would help us if the cause was not mechanical but some sort of infection so this is a good herb to start with that covers a lot of bases. For our antispasmodic herbs we will use Chamomile which has a strong antispasmodic action along with being loaded with magnesium and calcium which is what every screaming nerve needs. To back up

Chamomile we will add Passion Flower which is a pain killer, antispasmodic along with being a sedative and relaxant. Below is another herbal formula for this condition. If the problem is becoming a Chronic Condition go into the Herbal and look at the herb Shizandra.

Herbal Formula Sciatica
Rhus Tox 3X for pain relief
Jamaican dogwood - powerful sedative and anodyne
Oats - nerve tonic
Black cohosh - antispasmodic, sedative and anodyne
Valerian - sedative, hypnotic, antispasmodic
Black willow - anti-inflammatory, anodyne

Black Cohosh

Cimicfuga Racemosa
Actions - Emmenagogue, anti-spasmodic, nervine, alterative, sedative, tonic, anodyne, vasodilator.
Black Cohosh has a normalizing action on the balance of female sex hormones and may be safely used to regain normal hormonal activity that should give relief to Menopause symptoms. This would be the herb for you if you also suffered from rheumatism or arthritis. Has hormone balancing properties, ovarian cramps or cramping pain in the womb, used to regain normal hormone activity, good for hot flashes, muscular and neuralgic pains with a good example being Sciatica. Black Cohosh may also lower blood pressure, lower cholesterol, help with insomnia and help with tinnitus. Regarded as a relaxing nervine.
Doses- For tincture is 2-4mls 3 times a day, One and a half teaspoonful's for tea 3 times a day.
Cautions- Best taken with meals so as to avoid any chance of upsetting tummy. Allow up to 8 weeks to see benefits in menopausal problems and even then the full benefit of the herb may not be reached till 6 months' time. Antibiotics can reduce the effect of this herb.

Homoeopathic Remedies for Sciatica

Colocynth 6C to 30C – The most important remedy in Sciatica, corresponding to the worst cases. There are pains in the sciatic nerve extending to the knee or to the heel, worse from any motion, and especially aggravated by cold. The pain is paroxysmal, followed by numbness and partial paralysis. There is a sensation which has been described as if the thigh were bound with iron bands, or as though screwed in a vise. The muscles are fearfully tense and fixed. Particularly is the right side involved, and there are stitches during walking. There is a sense of constriction around the hip. The pains, too, may come suddenly and leave suddenly; they may be sticking and burning, and all are worse from cold or damp and at night, when the patient can find no easy position for the limb.

Gnaphalium 6C to 30C – This remedy is quite similar to Colocynthis. It has intense neuralgic pains along the nerve, and numbness. The whole trunk and the main branches seem affected, worse when lying down, worse from motion, stepping and better while sitting in a chair. The pains extend to the toes.

Arsenicum 6C to 30C – With this remedy the pain is marked by complete intermissions. It exacerbates every night at a particular hour, and becomes unbearable. It is increased by vigorous and relieved by gentle motion. It is aggravated by cold, but relieved momentarily by warmth. It is a pure neuralgia, neither inflammatory, toxaemic nor reflex. Arsenicum is one of our most reliable remedies in sciatica. Chamomilla should also be thought of in pure neuralgias of the sciatic nerve with unbearable pains, and the more it pains the hotter the patient becomes.

Rhus Toxicodendron – This remedy typifies sciatica with muscular and ligamentous involvement. It is seldom adapted to recent cases, but comes in later. The pains are tearing and burning, worse during rest, alleviated a short time only during motion. There is lameness and a disposition to muscular twitching and the bowels are constipated. It is a rheumatic sciatica, the fibrous sheath of the nerve being involved. It is the best remedy for a combination of lumbago and sciatica. Sciatica arising from over-exposure to wet or from lifting, wrenching and over-exertion. Great relief from warmth.

Arnica is also a remedy for sciatica due to over-exertion. The acute pains are followed by a sensation as if bruised.

Ammonium Muriaticum 6C to 30C – Sciatica, with aggravation of pain while sitting, somewhat relieved by walking and entirely relieved by lying down. Pain in the left hip as if the tendons were too short. The legs feel contracted. Painful jerks, feet feel as if asleep.

Pulsatilla 6C to 30C – This remedy typifies a sciatica due to venous stasis and is useful in the milder forms where there is a sense of fatigue and heaviness, flying attacks, aching in loins and hips. Uterine sciatica. Here it is akin to such remedies as Sepia, Belladonna, Ferrum, Sulphur, Graphites and Mercurius.

Aconite 6C to 30C – The congestive variety of sciatica from exposure to colds, dampness and from suppressed perspiration indicates Aconite. There is much numbness, perverted sensation, pricking and a sense of coldness in the parts, especially toes. The pains are very severe and worse at night. The patient is restless; there is tingling along the affected nerve.

Belladonna 6C to 30C – Here the inflammation is high and the pains come on suddenly. There is a neuritis and the course of the nerve is sensitive; the pain is especially severe at night, the parts are sensitive to the touch, the least concussion or a draft of air aggravates. Severe lancinating pains coming on in the afternoon or evening; has to change position often; worse from motion, noise, shock or contact; cannot bear the clothing to touch him. Relieved by letting the limb hang down, warmth and the erect posture.

Nux Vomica 6C to 30C – From its action on the spinal cord, Nux is frequently the remedy in sciatica. It has lightning-like pains, with twitching of the parts. Violent pains and has to change position; pains shoot down into the foot, the limb is stiff and contracted and the parts feel paralyzed and cold. Better when lying on the affected side and from the application of hot water. Constipated bowels and sedentary habit.

Neuritis

Neuritis is Inflammation of a nerve or nerves usually associated with a degenerative process or disease with a good example being Shingles in the diseases and Diabetes which you could say is a degenerative process. Symptoms can be pain and tenderness, impaired sensation often with numbness or hypersensitivity, impaired strength such as in a limb and or reflexes and are usually confined to a specific portion of the body served by the inflamed nerve or nerves. Sometimes neuritis affects a specific nerve. Pain or partial paralysis along the course of the affected nerve could be the result of disease or pressure on or injury to the nerve. Wounds, lacerations and crush injuries in nerve rich areas such as the fingers, lips and knees are a good example of neuritis in trauma injuries and are a pain that we can all relate to. For these injuries we use the Herb St John's Wort also known as Hypericum. This is a very interesting herb with many hats which is one of the main First Aid herbs for injuries in nerve rich areas and especially for shooting pain down the nerves. It is an important and the main herb in Shingles used externally and internally not just for the pain but because it is an Anti-Viral focused on the nervous system, in Shingles we also use it in its lotion form or in a cream down the pathways of the nerves that are infected. In the past it was also used to stop Tetanus and recently it was finally admitted that it's as good as some antidepressants. Neuritis can be caused by compression of a nerve, contusion or trauma and by Vitamin B12 deficiency, B1 deficiency, Vitamin B6 excess, Physical injury, Infection, Herpes zoster also known as Shingles, Lyme Disease, Multiple Sclerosis, Guillain–Barré Syndrome, damage caused by Diabetes. **Herbal Treatment -** With Neuritis being such a general term you really have to find the cause which can be very difficult in some cases and obvious in others. St John's Wort is the specific for inflammation of the nerves with Chamomile and Valerian used as a support as they cover most of the Herbal Actions of the nervous system. Chamomile supplies lots of Calcium and Magnesium which is what a screaming and twitching nerve needs and is a strong antispasmodic. Consider the B Vitamins as they are water soluble and pass through the body very fast making highly coloured urine which is why lots of people are deficient in them. Do not wait too long before seeking medical help as badly damaged nerves sometimes never heal again. Read St John's Wort below which is our main First Aid remedy for Nerves.

Hypericum
(St John's Wort)

Actions- Anti-inflammatory, astringent, anti-viral, anti-spasmodic, nervine, vulnerary, antibacterial.

Taken internally has a sedative and pain reducing effect. For neuralgic pain, anxiety, tension, rheumatic pain, sciatica, for pains that shoot along the nerves, as a lotion it will speed the healing of wounds and bruises and is used where there is damage to the nerve rich areas, varicose veins and mild burns. Good for inflamed joints and rheumatic pain. Recently the herb has become popular to use as an antidepressant especially for cases of anxiety. For First Aid use we are concentrating on external use only. Used for wounds with pains that shoot along the nerves, in nerve rich areas such as the fingers, lips, tail bone and toes. As a lotion it will speed the healing of wounds and bruises and is used where there is nerve damage and the possibility of tetanus. The main remedy for puncture wounds. Good for, varicose veins especially the painful kind and mild burns. Patients recovering from surgery where the nerves have been damaged often recover faster with Hypericum. For inflamed joints and rheumatic pain, painful abscesses, bad insect stings, damaged nerves from impact injuries, sprains and ulcers. Eases the pain in conditions such as lumbago, sciatica and Shingles where a cream can be used on the sore and the oil applied along the affected nerve path. As a lotion it is commonly mixed with Calendula, Homoeopaths call this lotion Hypercal. **How To Use -** Use as a Lotion one part tincture to twenty parts water to wash out wounds or medicate affected area, make at 1 to 10 for painful and dirty wounds. Mix with Calendula in large painful bleeding wounds with a chance of tetanus. Use Tincture for medicating creams. **Dose -** 1 to 4mls 3 times a day.

Shingles

Shingles is a skin infection by the same virus that causes chickenpox but mostly effects people over 50 years of age with a weakened immune system, the virus is called the Varicella zoster virus. This is a virus of the nervous systems that usually travels out from the spine. Infection of the intercostal nerves has the infection following the nerves that travel around the trunk while infection further up the spine travels to the neck or face. The virus may spread from one or more ganglia along nerves of an affected segment and infect the corresponding dermatome (an area of skin supplied by one spinal nerve) causing a painful rash. Although the rash usually heals within two to four weeks, some sufferers experience residual nerve pain for months or years, a condition called post herpetic neuralgia. When the virus activates it travels along nerve fibres, usually breaking out on one side of the body into small blisters called vesicles. Within a few days the blisters rupture forming scabs. Shingles is associated with severe pain, itching, redness, numbness, and the development of a rash. Shingles can affect the eyes. This is due to the fact that the eyes are connected to nerves that may be infected with the virus. Early diagnosis and treatment is important to minimize the symptoms and reduce the risk of complications that may compromise vision.

The symptoms are of a painful red rash that develops into fluid-filled blisters that can take several weeks to settle. It can occur on all parts of the body. The key to avoiding shingles is to assure general good health, especially a strong immune system. People who have had chickenpox cannot "catch" shingles from someone who has it. However, people who've never had chickenpox can be infected with chickenpox if exposed to someone with an active case of shingles.

Prevention - Unlike chickenpox, you can't catch shingles from someone who has it. However, it can be spread if you come into contact with the fluid contained in the blisters via contact with lesions or dressings and clothing stained with the fluid. There is a vaccine for adults over 50 available on prescription. The rash sheds the varicella-zoster virus and can be contagious. A caregiver or other person who lacks immunity developed from a prior case of chickenpox or the vaccine must avoid coming into contact with the rash or contaminated materials. Keep away from unimmunised children.

Symptoms - At the onset of shingles there's an intense pain and a burning or tingling sensation on the skin along with a general feeling on being unwell. The rash usually takes the shape of a band around the body because the virus works down the nerves that branch out from the spinal cord and encircle the body and can be very painful. Although the rash starts as a group of small bumps they soon form fluid-filled blisters that break open to form a crusty surface. The rash can be so tender that even a breeze may cause pain and can last for a few days or weeks. Another good description is as follows. The first symptom is usually one-sided pain, tingling, or burning. The pain and burning may be severe. Red patches on the skin form, followed by small blisters that look very similar to early chickenpox. The blisters break, forming small ulcers that begin to dry and form crusts. The crusts fall off in 2 to 3 weeks. The rash usually involves a narrow area from the spine around to the front of the belly area or chest. It may involve face, eyes, mouth and ears. Additional symptoms may include, abdominal pain, chills, difficulty moving some of the muscles in the face, drooping eyelid, fever, a general ill-feeling , headache, hearing loss, joint pain, loss of eye motion , swollen glands (lymph nodes), taste problems, vision problems and severe neuralgic pains. The lesion develops 3 days after the onset of a attack starting as reddish plaques developing along the nerve pathway, which turn into crops of vesicles which speedily increase in size. The vesicles contain serous fluid which in a few days the contents become opaque. Absorption of the contents occurs and brown adherent crusts form. In few weeks crusts separate leaving pigmented scars. Regional lymph glands can become enlarged and painful. **Prognosis -** The pain often lasts from two to four weeks, but in some cases, it can last for months. If it does, you've moved from shingles to a condition known as post herpetic neuralgia. Complications can be blindness (if lesions occurs in the eye), deafness, post-herpetic neuralgia, secondary bacterial skin infections, Ramsay-hunt syndrome which can lead to loss of movement in the face, hearing loss, loss of taste, and other symptoms. **Treatment** - Anti-viral medication is most effective if administered within three days of the rash appearing. Some Doctors prescribe

Lysine to people with cold sores, shingles, and genital herpes. Cool wet compresses can help with the itch to prevent scratching and therefore scarring. Give a light but nutritious diet and ensure plenty of rest. **Herbal Treatment -** We need to boost the immune system and improve nutrition as these are a big part of the cause of the disease so we start with Echinacea. The next two herbs we add are Hypericum (St John's Wort) and Lemon Balm as these are both strong nervines with Hypericum being one of our best pain killers but their most important action that we are using them for is because they are Anti-Viral Nervines. These are taken internally but can also be applied directly to the affected area in a 1 to 10 lotion, frequently Liquorice is another to consider for the formula as it also has a Anti-Viral action along with Anti Inflammatory and Demulcent actions and has also been applied directly to the rash mixed with the others. Passion Flower can be used for reducing pain along with Red Pepper (see below). Consider Peppermint and Pennyroyal along with most of the peppermint family which have long been used for this condition. The herbs mentioned so far are the main and important ones for this condition but don't forget to treat symptoms as they arise with the appropriate herbs. Red pepper (Capsaicin) is one of the more powerful herbal remedies for shingles as it contains the ingredient that makes it hot called capsaicin. Capsaicin brings relief by blocking pain signals from nerves just under the skin. Test it on a small area of skin and remember the hotter it gets the better it can act as a nerve block. Discontinue if it causes irritation. Ask your Pharmacist for creams containing capsaicin.

Vitamin C

Below is a write up about Dr. Warnocks ideas on Vitamin C taken from the net. I tend to agree with what he says. Have a look in The Disease Fighting Supplements part at my write up about Vitamin C.

High doses of vitamin C have been shown to keep the varicella-zoster virus from replicating, according to some studies involving people who were given intravenous injections. There have not been any studies that showed similar effects from taking oral supplements. Dr. Warnock believes, however, that you can help keep the virus from taking hold with a daily dose of 10,000 milligrams of vitamin C. Dr.

Warnock recommends five doses of 2,000 milligrams each, taken three hours apart. "The dosage goes beyond being a simple immune booster," he says. "The point is to interrupt the virus." Dr. Warnock thinks vitamin C might prevent the virus from multiplying and spreading along the infected nerve. At the same time, vitamin C may ease inflammation in the nerve and lessen the outbreaks of the lesions, he says. With a dose this high, you might experience an upset stomach and diarrhoea, which is a frequent side effect of excess vitamin C. If so, just reduce the dose until you reach a level that's more tolerable, says Dr. Warnock. "Also, you need to take this treatment early in the infection," he says. "Once there are millions of virus particles floating around, it becomes a much harder task to keep them from reproducing."

B12 - Taken about 3 times a day throughout the infection may reduce pain and the time of the infection.

Echinacea

Echinacea angustifolia

Actions - Immune stimulant, anti-microbial, anti-inflammatory, alterative, healing.

This herb is an infection fighter active against strep bacteria (abscesses and boils), a blood cleanser, (blood poisons, snake bites, poisonous insects) and a glandular and lymphatic system cleanser. Use it particularly for respiratory infections and for any disease above the waist. This is one of our main immune boosters for the acute diseases. Echinacea stimulates the bone marrow to make more white blood cells which are our main infection killers and why we only use it in short bursts. Use as a prophylactic to protect from infections especially when traveling or before going into Hospital. **Uses** - All infections, depressed immune function, inflammatory conditions, allergies, effective against both bacteria and viruses. **Dose** – 1 to 4mls of tincture. **Warning** - Do not use continually as you will burn out the immune system give a few weeks break after 3 weeks. Beware also in the use of allergies for you could be building up the immune system just to attack it.

Homeopathic Treatment for Shingles

Arsenic 30C - Herpes typically affects the lips, the face and intercostal region. With the eruptions there are intense burning sensations in the blister. Patient is worse after midnight and from cold in any form. Patient feels better by warmth. Patient feels very thirsty and gets prostrated very easily. Herpetic eruptions alternate with internal affections. Great Prostration, with rapid sinking of the vital forces; fainting. There may be Depression, melancholy, despairing, indifference or they can be Anxious, fearful, restless, full of anguish or Irritable, sensitive, peevish, easily vexed. The greater the suffering the greater the anguish, restlessness and fear of death. Mentally restless, but physically too weak to move. This remedy is indicated by its periodicity and time aggravation: after mid-night, and from 1-2 a.m. And by its intense restlessness, mental and physical and its anxiety and prostration.

Calc Carb 30C - Adapted to persons with impaired nutrition and a disposition to always getting sick, and who have a tendency to grow fat; herpes with burning and jerking pains which are worse in cold at night. Herpes with thick corrosive scabs which have yellow pus beneath them. Suppressed herpes causes central nervous system disorders. Calc Carb suits the person with a Leucophlegmatic constitution, blond hair, light complexion, blue eyes, fair skin and a tendency to obesity in youth. Psoric constitutions, pale, weak, timid, easily tired when walking. Disposed to grow fat, corpulent, unwieldy. Curvature of bones, especially spine and long bones; extremities crooked, deformed; bones irregularly developed. Head sweats profusely while sleeping.

Causticum 30C - Herpetic eruptions on shoulders, neck, around nipples and chin, face. There is itching burning pain which is worse in open air, in clear fine weather and is better in damp weather and from walking. Adapted to persons with dark hair and rigid fibre; weakly, psoric, with excessively yellow, sallow complexion; subject to affections of respiratory and urinary tracts.

Graphites 30C - Has a special affinity for folds of skin, e.g. joints, behind ears, groins, neck. Herpes in obese females with delayed and scanty menses. Herpes appearing at climateric. Large blisters from umbilicus to the spine, mainly affecting left side. Itching spots on various parts of the body which oozes a watery sticky fluid. Itching as though foreign matter would pass out through the skin. Circular herpes, feels hard to touch and is wrinkled. The itching is worse at night, during and after menstruation and is better from wrapping up. Suited to - Excessive cautiousness; timid, hesitates; unable to decide about anything. Fidgety while sitting at work. Sad, despondent; music makes her weep; thinks of nothing but death.

Hepar Sulph 30C - Face, hands, genitals and bends of knees and elbows are the commonly affected regions. Herpes after abuse of mercury. Adapted to persons with unhealthy skin which suppurates easily. Patients are highly sensitive to cold. Herpes zoster from spine forwards, especially the left side. The eruption is the seat of acute neuralgic pains which are worse at night; vesicles on an inflamed base associated with splinter like pains, severe itching and scratching. There is marked aggravation at night, from cold; touch and the patient feels better in damp weather and from wrapping up warmly. Especially suited to persons with a sour body odour. For sluggish and inactive lymphatic constitutions; persons with light hair and complexion, slow to act, muscles soft and flabby. The slightest injury causes suppuration. Diseases where the system has been injured by the abuse of Mercury. In diseases where suppuration seems inevitable, Hepar may open the abscess and hasten the cure. Oversensitive, physically and mentally; the slightest cause irritates him; quick, hasty speech and hasty drinking. Patient is peevish, angry at the least trifle; hypochondriacal; unreasonably anxious. Extremely sensitive to cold air, imagines he can feel the air if a door is opened in the next room; must be wrapped up to the face even in hot weather; cannot bear to be uncovered; takes cold from slightest exposure to fresh air.

Mercurius Sol 30C - Has a marked affinity for right side. Herpes of right forearm, wrist & hand. Herpes prepucialis of the right side extending across the abdomen. There is itching which changes to burning on scratching & shooting pains which are worse at night & in cold damp weather. Herpetic eruptions which are surrounded by small pimples. Herpes with a tendency to suppurate especially in persons with profuse sweat. Nervous affections after suppressed discharges especially in psoric patients. Glandular and scrofulous affections of children.

Mezereum 30C - Herpes following the intercostal or supraorbital nerves with severe neuralgia; itching after scratching turns into burning. Itching worse in bed & from touch. Post herpatic neuralgia & burning with great coldness of body. Herpes tends to ulcerate & forms thick scabs under which purulent matter exudes; tearing of these scabs causes great pain & retards healing. Herpes after suppressed eruptions; vaccination & abuse of mercury. For light-haired, irresolute persons of a phlegmatic temperament. Eczema and itching eruptions after vaccination. Hypochondriacal and despondent; indifferent to everything and everyone; angry at trifles and perfectly harmless things, but is soon sorry for it.

Ranunculus Bulbosus 30C - Herpes affecting the supraorbital & intercostal nerves. There are sharp stitching pains which are worse from touch, motion, change of temperature & on entering a cold place. The vesicles are filled with a thin, acrid fluid & are found in clusters. Herpetic eruptions over fingers & palms of hands which finally spreads over the whole body. Herpes in drunkards. One of our most effective remedies for the bad effects of alcoholic beverages; spasmodic hiccough; delirium tremens. Day blindness; mist before eyes, pressure and smarting in eyeballs.

Rhus Tox 30C - Herpes with a marked predilection for the right side & hairy parts. Herpes of the face. The itching is worse in winter & while sweating. Itching alternates with pains in the chest & dysenteric stools. Adapted to persons of rheumatic diathesis; bad effects of getting wet, especially after being over-heated. "Worse cold, wet". Worse wet; bathing; washing; strain. Drawing, tearing pain, especially fibrous tissues; joints; round joints. Restlessness; must move, though first movement painful. Better from dry, warm application.

Silica 30C - Dry herpes affecting the chin. Eruptions are inclined to suppurate. Suited to malnourished persons with unhealthy easily suppurating skin. Adapted to the nervous, irritable, sanguine temperament; persons of a psoric diathesis. Persons of light complexion; fine dry skin; pale face; weakly, with lax muscles. Constitutions which suffer from deficient nutrition, not because food is lacking in quality or quantity, but from imperfect assimilation; oversensitive, physically and mentally.

Sulphur 30C - Dry scaly herpes on nape of neck & ankles. Moist herpes with small white vesicles in groups, forming scabs over the whole face, especially above nose & about the eyes. There is burning pain after scratching. The patient is always worse from washing, bathing.

Adapted to persons of a scrofulous diathesis, subject to venous congestion; especially of portal system. Persons of nervous temperament, quick motioned, quick tempered, plethoric, skin excessively sensitive to atmospheric changes. For lean, stoop-shouldered persons who walk and sit stooping like old men. Standing is the worst position for sulphur patients; they cannot stand; every standing position is uncomfortable. Dirty, filthy people, prone to skin affections. Aversion to being washed; always worse after a bath. Too lazy to rouse himself; too unhappy to live.

Covering Headaches ending at Meningitis

Here we go through the different types of headaches which hopefully we can stop at the beginning. Concentrate on the causes with the most common one being stress.

Headaches
Try these First for Relief and Reducing Them

Dehydration – Can cause headaches. Thick blood is harder to move and pump so water it down and make the blood vessels happier. If you have problems with headaches and think this may be a cause go to a health shop that sells sports supplements and buy a couple of sachets Magnesium rehydration formula (racing bike riders use them) and see what happens as Magnesium can also give fast relief for headaches at the beginning.

B Vitamins - The B Vitamins stimulate the immune system, help in the regulation of the metabolism and the formation of neurotransmitters, such as serotonin, which may be deficient in people who suffer from migraines. The B vitamins are all water soluble, and a lot of you may have noticed that after you have taken them, the next time you urinate the urine will have taken on a fluorescent color which is all the B vitamins which have not been assimilated escaping. That's the problem with the Bs they don't stay for long but are always needed. I have put this next to dehydration so you can consider the damage being done by having reduced water which would slow down these vitamins in their important work; you would be affecting nearly every system in the body. B2 may reduce the frequency and duration of migraines; vitamin B3 calms vascular headaches by opening up blood vessels to increase blood flow. Stress rapidly reduces B vitamins along with magnesium and calcium.

Magnesium Citrate - Citrate means that it is water soluble so you will absorb it faster. Those who suffer from serious headaches often have low levels of magnesium. Magnesium also alleviates irritability, fatigue, blood pressure, and depression. This mineral is often deficient in people who consume a diet high in refined carbohydrates and sugar. Such diets deplete the body of the minerals chromium, manganese, zinc and the B complex vitamins. Taking 200–600 mg of magnesium a day can help reduce the frequency of headache attacks.

Food Sources - Lettuce, garlic, tomatoes, potatoes, raisins, bananas, almonds, cashews, dates, most whole grains, wheat germ, spinach, peas, celery.

Common Four Types of Headaches

Tension and Stress - This is the most common type of headache also known as stress headaches. These are the kind of non-progressive headaches causing mild to moderate pain and are usually non progressive, so get up and do something else for a while and get away from the stress and it may go away. **Herbs** to think of are Chamomile tea as it is loaded with magnesium and easy to find. If that fails go to Valerian. Try a relaxing bath with Essential oils of Lavender, Rosemary and Peppermint. They can also be rubbed on the forehead and temples.

Chamomile
Matricaria recutita
Actions - Antispasmodic, nervine, sedative, carminative, anti-inflammatory, analgesic, antiseptic, allergies.

An excellent gentle sedative with a relaxing action that is good for easing anxiety and helping with sleep. Helps to restore the nervous system. It is safe to use in children and is a powerful anti-inflammatory in almost any condition and a good all round tonic for the nervous system. This is the herb for those that can worry themselves sick. As a relaxant, chamomile depresses the central nervous system, reducing anxiety while not disrupting normal performance or function. Chamomile has been used for centuries to lower pain and reduce inflammation. This seems to be backed up by science with a 2009 study finding that chamomile caused cell reactions similar to that of nonsteroidal anti-inflammatory drugs. In the digestive system it can be used for indigestion especially when there are colicky pains and is ideal for colitis and IBS type problems. For females Chamomile is good for amenorrhea, spasmodic dysmenorrhea, premenstrual irritability and menopausal tensions. This herb is also a good source of calcium and magnesium which are the nervous systems favorite minerals. **Uses** - Anxiety, colic, diverticula's, flatulence, gastritis, indigestion, insomnia, irritable, nervousness, restlessness, stress, ulcers.

Doses - Tincture 2 to 4mls 3 times daily, for teas just the one teabag.

Hormonal Problems - Herbs that are good for balancing of the hormonal system. **Herbs** - Black Cohosh, Chaste Tree, Life Root, False Unicorn Root or Skullcap may help.

Skullcap
Scutellaria laterifolia
Action - Sedative, anti convulsive, tonic, nervine, antispasmodic, anodyne, hypotensive and anticonvulsant, stress, anxiety, PMS, anti depressive, alterative.

Skullcap has a wide range of use mostly focusing on the nerves and is a nervous system relaxant and tonic. Relaxes nervous tension while helping to strengthen the central nervous system and can be used for a wide range of conditions. Good for long term exhaustion and nervous tension. Has a specific use in the treatment of seizures and hysterical states along with epilepsy, muscular twitching, tremors and neuralgias. Used for all exhausted states and depressed conditions. Good for easing premenstrual and painful menstruation conditions due to its sedative and antispasmodic action. Use for weakness of the heart, irregular cardiac action, nervous irritation and physical exhaustion and insomnia. Skullcap eases the symptoms of drug and alcohol withdrawal such as muscle aches, shakiness, twitches, digestive distress, agitation, and poor quality sleep. Once the crisis is over Skullcap can decrease cravings for addictive substances. **Part used** - Aerial parts. **Precautions** - Avoid with tranquilisers or sedatives as Skullcap is a sedative in its own right and probably more balanced. **Combinations -** It combines well with Valerian. **Dosage-** Tincture 2 to 4mls 3 times daily. Infusion 1 to 2 teaspoons full of dried herb infused for 10 minutes.

Blood Pressure - These are more related to the Tension and Stress headaches but the herbs I mention here will also help with the Hormone headaches. **Herbs** are Mistletoe and Lime Flowers.

Mistletoe
Viscum album
Actions - Cardiac tonic, hypotensive, diuretic, antispasmodic, peripheral dilator, cardiac depressant, blood pressure normalizer, sedative, antitumor, anti-inflammatory, immune enhancer, has nervine properties on vascular system. **Uses** - Specific for arterial hypertension, arteriolosclerosis, nervous tachycardia, hypertensive headaches, hypertrophy of the heart with valvular insufficiency, dropsy of the extremities, weak pulse and labored breathing, has a wide application for treating nervous diseases, reduces bleeding. The Herbalist David Hoffman says *"Mistletoe opens up circulation to areas that have been cut off from adequate blood supply by tension. It reduces cardiovascular tension and blood pressure, while bringing in new blood, blood sugar, and healing to areas long cut off, tensed up, weakened, or damaged."* Reduces the symptoms of high blood pressure, particularly headaches and dizziness. Good for anxiety and panic attack as Mistletoe acts to lower the stress hormone cortisol, bringing the nerves down to a more manageable level. Improves concentration, insomnia, tinnitus and epilepsy. Soothes and tones the nervous

system, acts directly on the vagus nerve to reduce heart rate whilst strengthening the wall of the peripheral capillaries. Useful for nervous tachycardia and headaches from high blood pressure. Mistletoe has been used traditionally as a relaxant and herbal remedy for sleep for centuries. Mistletoe is also now being considered immune stimulant which can stimulate and modulate the immune system. **Precautions** – Pregnancy and not for children. May clash with some medications. **Combinations** - Combines well with Hawthorn Berries and Lime Blossom in the treatment of high blood pressure. **Contra Indications** - Berries are toxic. **Dose** – 1 to 3mls of tincture 3 times daily. Infusion 1 to 2 teaspoon full to cup of boiling water.

Migraine - After this section there will be a full write up on Migraine Headaches, the herb below can sometimes abort or reduce the headache. Migraines can last from a few hours to a few days and usually have other symptoms such as sensitivity to light, noise or smells, blurry vision, nausea and or vomiting and sometimes extreme pain that may last for a long time, with the patient preferring a darkened room. **Causes** – Seem to occur due to a combination of nerve signals sent from the blood vessels and muscles in the head. Exact causes are not known but obvious ones can be stress, dehydration, too much sun, excessive noise, eyestrain, smoke, chemicals, paints, perfumes, medical conditions such as high blood pressure, sinus, tumour, fever, or run in the family, allergies especially from food sensitivities.

Lime Flower

Tilia europea

Actions - Nervine, antispasmodic, hypotensive, diaphoretic, diuretic, sedative, mild astringent, anti-inflammatory, peripheral vasodilator, anti-coagulant.

Possesses powerful nerve and blood cleansing properties, used for fits and nervous twitching of all kinds including epilepsy, nervous tension, as a prophylactic against arteriosclerosis, migraines, feverish colds and flu. It is hypotensive; although it is rarely strong enough on its own to reduce blood pressure, it will reduce hypertension when associated with arteriosclerosis and nervous tension. Indicated in hysterical states, headaches, palpitations and nervous dyspepsia. Also notable as a diaphoretic (reduces fevers) and is often used in colds and flu. **Heart Health** - Used for atherosclerosis when the arteries lose their flexibility and elasticity which is the main cause of heart disease. Linden helps to maintain the smooth inner surface and elasticity of the blood vessel walls. One of the active ingredients in Linden is an essential oil called farnesol which acts as a sedative helping to relax the cardiovascular system which in turn helps to curb stress and anxiety. **Respiratory System** - The main uses of Lime Flowers in the past was to treat coughs, colds and the flu. It contains mucilage which soothes the irritated membranes of the throat and it is known to decrease mucus production. Lime Flowers are rich in antioxidant flavonoids and anti-inflammatory compounds that can help to reduce cold and flu symptoms such as inflamed membranes in the respiratory tract. Being a diaphoretic it can help if a cold or the flu turns into a fever by inducing a bout of sweating which can often break the fever. **Digestion** - Acts as a carminative herb and bitter tonic that can be used to aid a digestive upset especially in the tea form. Can stimulate digestion while reducing gastrointestinal discomfort. Linden tea can be especially useful for excessive gas causing the stomach to push up and put pressure on the heart. The anti-spasmodic action of Lime Flowers works by relieving spasms in the intestinal tract. **Uses** - Treatment of all nervous ailments especially epilepsy, twitching, vertigo, good for colds and to remove mucous from the system, treatment of vomiting, heart pains, fevers and the treatment of tumors by poultice.

Dose - 1 to 2mls of tincture 3 times a day. Tea, 1 teaspoon full infused in a cup 3 to 5 times a day.

Homoeopathic Remedies for Headaches

Belladonna 6 to 30C - Belladonna is the first remedy that comes to mind in headache; its symptoms are clear and sharply defined. Throbbing is the great keynote, but violent shooting pains in the head, driving the patient almost wild, are scarcely less characteristic. The patient cannot lie down, must sit up, nor can they bear light, a draft of air, noise or jarring; this last is most characteristic. The location of the ache is mostly in the frontal region or right side, flushed face, dilated pupils accompany. Glonoine is the only remedy having throbbing as characteristic as Belladonna. Glonoine, however, does not have such a lasting effect as Belladonna; it is more relieved by motion, the face is not so deeply flushed, and there is aggravation from bending the head backwards, and it has the explosive bursting characteristic of nitro-glycerine; all of which will serve to distinguish the two remedies; it has the feeling of a tight band across the forehead. Its curative action is rapid. Cinchona also has throbbing, but here it is due to anaemia. Belladonna has also a symptom common to Nux vomica and Bryonia, namely, a feeling as if the head would burst. The headaches of Belladonna are usually worse in the afternoon, the whites of eyes are red, and the cornea is glassy, and moving eyes aggravates. The face is puffed and red.

Nux vomica 6 to 30C - It is quite safe to assert that Nux vomica is more often indicated in headache than any other remedy; this is presumably due in the main to the cause of headache calling for Nux vomica; thus, we have the headache from the excessive use of alcohol, the morning "big head," tobacco, coffee, headache from digestive troubles, constipation, and specially auto- "intoxication" and hepatic insufficiency. These are all common causes of the Nux vomica headache. It suits the gouty and Haemorrhoidal, which makes up four-fifths of all migraines. The ache is situated over one or the other eye, usually the left, or else in the occiput. It is apt to being in the morning with giddiness on first rising, and last all day until night, and is accompanied with sour taste or perhaps nausea and violent retching. The dull, wooden, bursting feeling of the head following a debauch is most characteristic of Nux vomica. Headaches of high livers call for Nux. The complexion looks muddy and the whites of the eyes are yellow, and the urine is scanty and high colored. Jousset recommends the 12X or 30X between attacks. There are some modalities of the Nux vomica headache that should be carefully noted, as this point will sometimes aid greatly in making a selection; for instance: Stooping and coughing aggravate the headache; it is worse in the morning; moving the eyes and motion in general makes the head feel worse. What relieves the Nux vomica headache is not so clear; certain headaches calling for Nux will be better by wrapping the head up warm and by rest, but these conditions are rare ones calling for the drug. In general, nothing relieves the Nux vomica headache; but it will often disappear by rising and being about for a few hours. This is a characteristic point in those headache due to alcoholic excesses. A headache "all over the head" is also characteristic of Nux.

Sanguinaria 6 to 30C - Genuine sick headache calls for this drug, and the symptoms in brief are these: The pain begins in the morning and in the occiput; it comes up over the head and settles in the right eye. The pain increases in severity until there is vomiting of food and bile, then oftentimes the ache is relieved, will be so intense at times that the patient will frantically bore her headache into the pillow for relief. It is especially suitable to women who menstruate too freely. Belladonna may easily be differentiated by the following points: It has hot head, more throbbing, flushed face and cold feet, and the pain coming up from the occiput is not so marked as under Sanguinaria. The Sanguinaria headache is relieved by lying down, Belladonna by being propped up in bed, and Sanguinaria is more useful in the gastric form of headache. There may be also profuse micturition with Sanguinaria relieving the headache, as we find under Gelsemium, Ignatia and in a less degree under some other drugs.

Iris Versicolor 6 to 30C - The Iris headache characteristically commences with a partial blindness, or blurring of vision, being similar here to Gelsemium and Kali bichromicum, and it is especially a remedy for gastric or bilious headaches. This blurring of the sight may be preceded by drowsiness and the head begins to ache as soon as the blurring disappears. It is useful remedy for Sunday headache, not, however, in that form which sometimes occur as a convenient excuse for non-church attendance (which is incurable), but that form which occurs in teachers, scholars, professors, etc., in whom a relief of the strain of the preceding six days produces the headache. The pains are mostly located over the eyes in the supra-orbital ridges, usually in one side at a time, mostly the right. The dental nerves are frequently affected. The pains are throbbing or sharp, and when at their acme vomiting occurs, which is apt to be copious, bitter or sour. Especially characteristic is vomiting of matters so sour that the teeth are set on edge. The headache of Iris is aggravated by violent motion, cold air and coughing; moderate exercise in the open air relieves. In sick headache with continuous nausea it is one of our most useful remedies, and if indicated closely by the above symptoms it will not fail. When headaches are produced by eating sweet things Iris is probably the remedy.

Migraine Headaches

Migraine headaches are caused by the combination of the chemicals released from nerve fibres that coil around the blood vessels and vasodilatation (widening of the blood vessels). The chemicals cause inflammation, further enlargement of the artery and pain. Migraine headache patients are typically smart, inflexible and disciplined. Sudden migraine attacks may occur due to overworked muscles in the head and neck and due to continuous stress. The blood flow drops because these tight muscles squeeze the arteries. When the person suddenly relaxes these tight muscles expand and stretch the blood vessel walls. The blood pumped with each heartbeat then pushes the vessels further causing immense pain. A migraine is usually an intense pounding headache with nausea that occurs from time to time. The pounding or pulsing pain usually begins in the forehead, the side of the head or around the eyes. The headache gradually gets worse. Bright lights or loud noises make the headache worse. Genetics and environmental factors are considered to be the causes of migraines. Imbalances in brain chemicals are thought to be involved. Serotonin levels which help to regulate in the nervous system drop during a migraine. This effect causes the trigeminal system to release neuropeptides which are sent to the meninges of the brain resulting in headache pain. Symptoms typically last 4 to 72 hours and may be severe. Pain is often unilateral, throbbing, worse with exertion, and accompanied by symptoms such as nausea and sensitivity to light, sound, or odours. Auras occur in about 25% of patients, usually just before but sometimes after the headache. Migraine triggers include hormonal changes, various foods, stress, physical activity, environmental changes, some medications and some sensory stimulants such as flashing lights, smells of certain odours like cigarette smoke or perfumes. Migraine can affect adults and children as well. Before puberty, the ratio that suffers from migraine in boys and girls remain same, but after adolescence women suffer more than men.

Migraine is often wrongly diagnosed with sinus or tension headaches.

Compared To Other Headaches

Migraine Headaches - In the migraine headache there are recurrent attacks. They are described as throbbing, intense and pounding pain that involve one side of the head known as temple. Sometimes they may involve the forehead, around eyes or the back of the head. The pain is generally unilateral and may change side to side. The attack is aggravated by climbing stairs, looking at sun and bending forwards. The symptoms include nausea, vomiting, sometimes diarrhoea, cold feet, sensitivity to light and sound and facial pallor. Migraine sufferers like to be in a quiet and dark room during an attack.

Tension Headaches - In tension headaches, the pain begins in the back of the head and upper neck as tightness or pressure like feeling. This headache is also described as a band of pressure encircling the entire head especially over eyebrows. They are seldom associated with vomiting, nausea or sensitivity to light and sound. 90% of adults have had or will have tension headaches. These types of headaches are more common in women compared to men.

Secondary Headaches - With these the cause is known for example from a stroke, sinus, tumour, meningitis, heatstroke flu etc.

Diagnosis - Diagnosis is based on characteristic symptoms and a normal physical examination, which includes a thorough neurologic examination. **Prevention** - Potential migraine triggers can be, drinking red wine, skipping meals, excessive stimuli (eg, flashing lights, strong odours), weather changes, sleep deprivation, stress, hormonal factors, head trauma, neck pain and many other things. Patients should to keep a written headache diary to document the number and timing of attacks, possible triggers, and response to treatment. **Prognosis** - For some patients, migraine is an infrequent, tolerable inconvenience. For others, it is a devastating disorder resulting in frequent periods of incapacity, loss of productivity, and severely impaired quality of life. Not enough is really understood so it is very important for those severely affected to keep a headache diary. **Symptoms -** Approximately 20 percent of people with migraines experience what's called an aura prior to the migraine, they last minutes to an hour. Symptoms of an aura include flashes of light, zig zags, or blind spots in your vision or tingling in one arm or leg, this is not an all-inclusive list as every person is individually different. Others experience drowsiness, thirst, depression or irritability. Other symptoms are moderate to severe pain on one or both sides of the head, Pulsating or pounding pain on one side of your head (or both), Pain worse with physical activity, nausea with or without vomiting, sensitivity to light, noise, and movement especially bending over which makes your head hurt and worse. Patients want to lie down in a dark, quiet room. There is no predictable migraine attack cycle that has been established yet. Migraines and depression are sometimes related in some persons. Headache varies from moderate to severe, and attacks last from 4 hours to several days, typically resolving with sleep. Keeping a Headache Diary is the main way in which to get a diagnosis from a Doctor. **Herbal Treatment -** The herb Feverfew is one of the main remedies for migraine and has been used for centuries as a remedy for headache, migraine, arthritis, pain, and fever in Europe. Feverfew is used as a preventative for migraines. This is achieved by taking a small dose of feverfew daily (125mg leaf). Feverfew contains parthenolide, a substance that inhibits the brain chemicals that dilate blood vessels and cause migraine. It has some of the same anti-inflammatory effects as aspirin but without the side effects. However, feverfew does need to be taken for several weeks before the effects are felt, so it is best used as a preventative measure. Do not come off Feverfew abruptly after taking it for a long time reduce dosage and go slow and do not use this herb if you are using blood thinking medication. I have found that Co Enzyme Q 10 at about 300mg can sometimes abort migraines if given at the right time when you have your first suspicions that this may be happening, if nothing happens follow up with some Gingko

Biloba which is a peripheral vasodilator mainly for the head and feet which we use to get herbs or in this case Q10 into these areas. Gingko Biloba by itself can be of help by opening up the arteries in the neck and restoring normal blood flow and can help to prevent migraine due to it can inhibit the platelet activating factor in the blood. Ginger (Zingiber officinale) contains constituents that inhibit platelet aggregation. Ginger tea works, for a migraine headache in the front of the head. Some have also reported as a good preventative. You can also buy Ginger in its crystallized form ranging from mild to really strong and this can be a fast and easy way to dose yourself. You can add to a formula Valerian which is more for stress headaches, while Damiana, Kola, Sarsaparilla and Ginseng are more for fatigue lassitude and general debility. Below are some other Herbal Formulas' used by well-known Herbalists.

Mittons Formula
Skullcap 45mgs
Lupulus 45
Gum Asafoetida 30
Aqueous extract of gentian 85
Valerian 100

Hoffmann
Black willow - analgesic, bitter, nervine tonic
Wood Betony - specific for head, tonic, bitter
Black horehound - anti emetic, sedative
Meadowsweet - GIT normaliser
Oats - nerve tonic
Skullcap - sedative, nervine
Ginseng - if stress induced

Webb's formula
Wood betony 30g
Rosemary 15
Skullcap 15
Infuse in 1.2 l of boiling water for 20 minutes, strain, Take 50mls 3 or

4 times daily.

Feverfew

Tanacetum parthenium

Actions - Analgesic, anti-inflammatory, emmenagogue, vasodilator, relaxant, digestive bitter, febrifuge, uterine stimulant.

Alleviates pain, headaches and inflammation and is similar to aspirin but stronger with a slower effect. Research has shown that feverfew inhibits the release of histamine from mast cells and inhibits the production of leukotrienes. Decreases inflammation in blood vessels and in arthritic conditions as well as increases menstrual flow and induces menstruation. The bitters stimulate appetite and improve digestion and kidney function. One of the main remedies used for migraines, especially those that are relieved by applying warmth to the head. Feverfew contains a chemical called parthenolide which helps relieve smooth muscle spasms and can combat the widening of blood vessels that occurs in migraines. Feverfew can reduce the frequency of migraines and reduce symptoms such as nausea, vomiting and sensitivity to light.

The bitters in Feverfew stimulate appetite and improve digestion. It is one of the most important aids for female ailments especially in menstrual cramps which occur when the lining of the uterus makes large amounts of prostaglandins when breaking these cells down during menstruation, the prostaglandins are released constricting the blood vessels in the uterus causing painful cramps. Increases menstrual flow and induces menstruation. Feverfews anti-inflammatory actions help to prevent swelling and damage to the joints in arthritis. **Contraindications** - Pregnancy due to emmenagogue effects. **Interactions** - May interfere with anti-coagulant medications. **Dose** - 3 to 4mls of tincture 3 times daily. For tablets take dosage on pack.

Nutrition

Migraine relief using B3 Niacin - Niacin has proved helpful in relieving migraine pain. Valuable sources of this vitamin are yeast, whole wheat, green leafy vegetables, tomatoes, nuts, sunflower seeds, liver and fish.

Magnesium - Several studies have evaluated the effectiveness of magnesium for migraine and have had promising results. In one study, oral magnesium (600 mg per day) or a placebo were given to 81 people with migraines. After nine weeks, the frequency of migraines was reduced by 41.6 percent in the group taking magnesium, compared to 15.8 percent in the group taking the placebo. The only reported side effects were diarrhoea in 18.6 percent of people and digestive irritation in 4.7 percent. Magnesium has many important uses for preventing migraines. Some of them are maintaining and improving blood vessel health, reducing sleep disorders, maintaining nerve and muscle function, decreasing blood coagulation and reducing blood pressure and normalizing heart rhythm.

Homoeopathic Treatment for Migraines

Belladonna 30C - Is the first remedy that comes to mind in headache; its symptoms are clear and sharply defined. Throbbing is the great keynote. The patient cannot lie down, must sit up, nor can he bear light, a draft of air, noise or jarring; this last is most characteristic. The location of the ache is mostly in the frontal region or right side, flushed face, dilated pupils accompany. Glonoine is the only remedy having throbbing as characteristic as Belladonna. Glonoine, however, does not have such a lasting effect as Belladonna; it is more relieved by motion, the face is not so deeply flushed, and there is aggravation from bending the head backwards, and it has the explosive bursting characteristic of nitro-glycerine; all of which will serve to distinguish the two remedies; it has the feeling of a tight band across the forehead. Its curative action is rapid. Cinchona also has throbbing, but here it is due to anaemia. Belladonna has also a symptom common to Nux vomica and Bryonia, namely, a feeling as if the head would burst. The headaches of Belladonna are usually worse in the afternoon, the whites of eyes are red, and the cornea is glassy, and moving eyes aggravates.

Nux Vom 30C - It is quite safe to assert that Nux vomica is more often indicated in headache than any other remedy. It suits the gouty and haemorrhoidal, which makes up four-fifths of all migraines. The ache is situated over one or the other eye, usually the left, or else in the occiput. It is apt to being in the morning with giddiness on first rising, and last all day until night, and is accompanied with sour taste or perhaps nausea and violent retching. The dull, wooden, bursting feeling of the head following a debauch is most characteristic of Nux vomica. Headaches of high livers call for Nux. The complexion looks muddy and the whites of the eyes are yellow, and the urine is scanty and high colour. There are some modalities of the Nux vomica headache that should be carefully noted, as this point will sometimes aid greatly in making a selection; for instance: Stooping and coughing aggravate the headache; it is worse in the morning; moving the eyes and motion in general makes the head feel worse. What relieves the Nux vomica headache is not so clear; certain headaches calling for Nux will be better by wrapping the head up warm and by rest, but these conditions are rare ones calling for the drug. In general, nothing relieves the Nux vomica headache; but it will often disappear by rising and being about for a few hours. This is a characteristic point in those headaches due to alcoholic excesses. A headache "all over the head" is also characteristic of Nux. Ptelea trifoliata. Dr. Kopp holds this remedy without a rival in frontal headaches,and it will often cure after other remedies have failed.

Sanguinaria 30C - Genuine sick headache calls for this drug, and the symptoms in brief are these: The pain begins in the morning and in the occiput; it comes up over the head and settles in the right eye. The pain increases in severity until there is vomiting of food and bile, then oftentimes the ache is relieved will be so intense at times that the patient will frantically bore her headache into the pillow for relief. It is especially suitable to women who menstruate too freely. Belladonna may easily be differentiated by the following points: It has hot head, more throbbing, flushed face and cold feet, and the pain coming up from the occiput is not so marked as under Sanguinaria. The Sanguinaria headache is relieved by lying down, Belladonna by being propped up in bed, and Sanguinaria is more useful in the gastric form of headache. There may be also profuse micturition with Sanguinaria relieving the headache, as we find under Gelsemium, Ignatia and in a less degree under some other drugs.

Iris Versicolor 30C - The Iris headache characteristically commences with a partial blindness, or blurring of vision and it is especially a remedy for gastric or bilious headaches. This blurring of the sight may be preceded by drowsiness and the head begins to ache as soon as the blurring disappears. It is useful remedy for Sunday headache, not, however, in that form which sometimes occur as a convenient excuse for non-church attendance (which is incurable), but that form which occurs in teachers, scholars, professors, etc., in whom a relief of the strain of the preceding six days produces the headache. The pains are mostly located over the eyes in the supra-orbital ridges, usually in one side at a time, mostly the right. The dental nerves are frequently affected. The pains are throbbing or sharp, and when at their acme vomiting occurs, which is apt to be copious, bitter or sour. Especially characteristic is vomiting of matters so sour that the teeth are set on edge. The headache of Iris is aggravated by violent motion, cold air and coughing, open air relieves. In sick headache with continuous nausea it is one of our most useful remedies, and if indicated closely by the above symptoms it will not fail. When headaches are produced by eating sweet things Iris is probably the remedy.

Gelsemium 30C - Gelsemium is another remedy which has a headache commencing with blindness, and especially a remedy for headaches due to eye strain. The ache under Gelsemium commences in the occiput or nape of the neck, comes up over the head settles in the eye as in Sanguinaria. There is a feeling as if a band was about the head, the patient is dull and apathetic, and there is great soreness in the eye when moving them. Occipital headaches, which are dull and dragging, often find their remedy in Gelsemium. Gelsemium headaches are also relieved by sleep, and dizziness may accompany. A characteristic of Gelsemium is a sensation of a band around the head just above the ears. It also suits "tobacco headaches.

Spigelia 30C - This remedy holds about the same relation to the left side of the head that Sanguinaria does to the right side. The pains are neuralgic in character, settle over the left eye and they are apt to follow the course of the sun, beginning in the morning, reaching the acme at noon and subsiding at sunset. There is often a sensation as if the head were open along the vertex. Noises and jarring of the bed, as under Belladonna, aggravate the pain; stooping and change of weather also make the pain worse. The pure neuralgic character of the pain, and its left side preference, should lead to the remedy.

Cimicifuga 30C - This is another remedy for the neuralgic form of headache and it has some valuable symptoms. It corresponds to headache of students and those exhausted by fatigue. There is first a sensation as if the top of the head would fly off. There are sharp, lancinating pains in and over the eyes, shooting to the top of the head. The brain seems to move in waves, and there may be the symptoms of a sharp pain extending from the occiput to the frontal region, as if a bolt were driven through the head. Headaches which are reflex or dependent on some uterine irritation are met by this remedy. When there is a feeling as if the patient would go crazy it is especially indicated. Many of the pains begin in the occiput and shoot down the spine; there is a tendency to bend the head forward, which relieves somewhat.

Silicea 30C - Silicea is a very useful remedy in headache, but one not very often used. When a patient with a headache has her head tied up with a towel or handkerchief it will probably indicate one of two remedies. Argentum nitricum if the head be tied up tightly; here we have relief from pressure; and Silicea if the head is tied up simply to keep it warm. The headache of Silicea is nervous and caused by excessive mental exertion. The face is pale at the commencement of the headache, but gets flushed as the pain becomes intense; body is chilly. It is supra-orbital and worse over the right eye, the pains coming up from the back of the head. Noise, motion and jarring aggravate. Warmth relieves. The headache of Silicea like that of Ignatia and Gelsemium is relieved by copious urination. An additional indication for Silicea is an extreme sensitiveness of the scalp.

Natrum Muriaticum 30C - The headache of Natrum muriaticum is as if there were little hammers beatings in the skull, worse from moving the head or eyeballs. It comes on in the morning, is worse about 10 A.M. and is preceded by partial blindness. The headache generally centers around the region of the ear and runs up to the parietal bone or occiput, leaving a stiffness of the nape of the neck, profuse urination relieving.

Meningitis

Yes the elderly can get Meningitis, my Grandma got it a 65 in the 1980s and she was always very careful not to drink the local water when she was travelling but came undone by an ice cube in Mexico. A common cause of bacterial meningitis in the elderly is the bacteria Streptococcus pneumoniae which also causes pneumonia as well as ear and sinus infections. Others in the elderly are Neisseria meningitides and Listeria monocytogenes. Bacterial meningitis remains a highly lethal disease in older adults with mortality rates averaging over 20%. The symptoms can also be slightly different then seen in the young with fewer patients manifesting fever, neck stiffness, and headache. The bad news is Antibiotics don't work as well as they used to. For the fit and healthy at 50 you may be prone to all the causes. **Cause -** Meningitis is an inflammation of the meninges, the membranes that cover the brain and spinal cord. Meningococcus causes meningitis and septicemia. Meningitis and septicemia account for more than 90% of meningococcal infections. Transmission generally occurs via direct contact with respiratory secretions from a carrier. Carrier rates rise dramatically during epidemics. After invading the body Meningococcus causes meningitis and severe bacteremia in both children and adults. Children between 6 months and 3 years are the most frequently infected. Other high-risk groups include adolescents, military recruits and college freshmen living in dormitories. Infection or vaccination confers type-specific immunity. The disease is most common among children and those of early youth, but it attacks adults up to perhaps twenty years of age quite commonly. No age however is free from liability to attacks during an epidemic. **Disease Process -** Meningitis is usually caused by bacteria or viruses (viral meningitis is called aseptic meningitis). Less common causes include fungi, protozoa, and other parasites. Meningitis is a severe acute inflammatory disorder involving the meninges of the brain and spinal cord. The disease can be epidemic, endemic and sporadic in occurrence, characterized by an abrupt onset with chill, fever, headache, pain in the spinal column, stiffness and contraction of the muscles of the neck and back and in violent cases impairment of the brain and mental function, mild coma or delirium, dullness of the eyes and irregularly contracting pupils or pupils irresponsive to light. **Diagnosis -** Diagnosis is confirmed by culture. Guiding symptoms can be the rash, photophobia and stiff neck. **Prevention -** Isolate patient. Vaccination is recommended for military recruits and travelers to endemic areas. Close contacts of people with meningococcal disease are at increased risk of acquiring the disease and should receive a prophylactic antibiotic. Symptoms are usually severe and include headache, nausea, vomiting, photophobia, lethargy, rash, multiple organ failure and shock. Patients with meningitis frequently report fever, headache, and stiff neck. Other symptoms include nausea, vomiting, photophobia, and lethargy. A maculopapular or hemorrhagic petechial rash often appears soon after disease onset.

The Following Is From Herbalist Finley Ellingwood, M.D. 1910
The following is a far better description of the symptoms so I have added it here.

In the epidemic form, as a rule, there are no prodromes, the patient being suddenly stricken down, from previous good health. Usually there is a chill, which is almost immediately accompanied with headache and dizziness, with an abrupt development of fever. The temperature usually is not high, but severe cases will reach 104° F. and hold that point steadily, with but slight variations for from twenty-four to thirty-six hours. A temperature of 102.5° F. is more common and is usual with the milder cases or with those of slow development. In many cases there is no marked variation in the temperature, often there is no change for a long period, but a reduction or increase of one degree perhaps within twelve or eighteen hours is not uncommon. The headache, which is one of the first symptoms, rapidly increases until it becomes almost unbearable.

This is accompanied with severe pain in the spinal cord, involving the muscles of the back. These muscles soon become rigid and the tenseness involves the muscles also of the thighs, arms and neck. Brain symptoms appear quickly, and consciousness is soon lost, the patient becoming dull and stupid and developing a mild delirium. In other cases the patient lies with the eyes open, but takes no notice of things around him and is soon found to be partially unconscious. In other cases there is great restlessness, with a high degree of nervous excitability. Commonly the stiffness occurs in the muscles of the back of the neck, the head is drawn backward and forced into the pillow, the head can be moved from side to side, but flexion and extension will result in excruciating pain, the posterior cervical muscles are hard and in a state of tonic contraction from irritation of the anterior roots of the cervical nerves The eruption of meningitis occurs in perhaps one-half of the sporadic or endemic cases. In epidemics it is present in the larger number of cases. The eruption by far the most common is the petechial eruption, from which the disease has the name of spotted fever. This occurs in the form of irregular purpuric spots, which may be diffused or limited to a small area. At first the eruption is quite red, later it occasionally becomes dark and appears as ecchymosis. To those who are experienced, the appearance of the eye assists greatly in diagnosis. Most commonly the eye is dull, with a dilated pupil. The eye may be very bright, with contracted pupil, or the pupils may be unequal in size, and in all cases not readily responsive to light. In the isolated cases, dullness of the mind, with somnolence, or stupor may occur early. In fatal cases this increases to coma, with no recurrence of consciousness. With the dullness there may be mild delirium, or nocturnal delirium only may occur, independent of any tendency to stupor. Active delirium with violent manifestations is not uncommon in the early stage. This may be accompanied with hallucinations, and in the female with hysterical manifestations. Vomiting is not an uncommon symptom. It is often of cerebral origin, but may be induced by faults of the stomach. The tongue is usually thick and pale, but slightly coated, and the appetite is early lost, but later the tongue becomes dark and dry, the secretions are all suppressed and sides appears. Constipation is apt to be present, with tympanic distension of the bowels.

At first the patient passes a large quantity of pale urine of low specific gravity. Later it is reduced in quantity, until but little is passed, which has a high specific gravity. Retention, suppression and incontinence are not uncommon during the later stages of the disease, and albumen and sugar are found in rare isolated cases.

Prognosis - Infection is associated with a mortality rate of 10 to 15%. Of patients who recover, 10 to 15% have serious sequelae, such as permanent hearing loss, mental retardation, or loss of phalanges or limbs. In Finley Ellingwoods time the death rate in severe epidemics was from fifty to seventy-five per cent. In mild epidemics from twenty to thirty per cent were fatal. In sporadic cases the mortality was very high, especially in young children. **Treatment** - Treatment is penicillin or a 3rd-generation cephalosporin. Corticosteroids decrease the incidence of neurologic complications in children. When corticosteroids are used, they should be administered with or before the 1st dose of antibiotics. Dexamethasone is given for 4 days. Ellingwood says the patient must be confined in an isolated room, away from confusion and noise of every kind, with a most careful and conscientious nurse, and the room should be darkened. The patient should receive a concentrated and highly nutritious diet. The disease is rapidly exhausting in its character and all measures must be adopted that will sustain the strength. Milk, eggs, beef juice, rice, and fruit juices must be given freely. When the active symptoms have abated, the physician should in no wise relax his assiduous attention, as the period of convalescence is apt to be long and recovery very slow. **Herbal Treatment** - This is another good example of beginning treatment before you know what the disease is because by the time you have figured this one out it is really too late to do that much. The herbs that Ellingwood was using in his time are far too dangerous for us to use now especially with our lack of experience with them for he was using them close to the toxic doses in serious diseases such as this. Safe specifics we can use that were used in the past are Baptisia, Boneset and Passion Flower for the pain. Basically concentrate on the strong Antibacterials especially those that work in and on the blood stream. As we should never really give up there is something else we can try. Essential Oils can cross what is known as the Blood Brain Barrier and get into the spinal fluid, now that we have that handy bit of information lets act upon it. First of all we will give heaps of Garlic oil internally in a serious case I would do it in 5 to 10 capsules of oil at a time. Next we will use a selection of Antibacterial and Antiseptic Essential Oils, choose from Tea Tree Oil, Garlic (puncture some Garlic Oil capsules), Eucalyptus, Rosemary, Lavender, Juniper, Bergamot and Sandalwood. Mix your formula with a carrier oil and apply to the neck and down the spine area till about the top of the hips. Essential Oils work by medicating the blood stream via the skin so care must be taken not to overdo it as it throws a load on the liver whose job it is to detox the blood, this is why caution should always be used using Aromatherapy. In our case we are concentrating on the spine and neck trying to get the oil into the cerebrospinal fluid so it can travel to the meninges and have a direct Antibacterial Action. The reality is you need a Ambulance and immediate hospitalization for those of us lucky to have it.

Homoeopathic Treatment for Meningitis

Belladonna 6C to 30C - Corresponds to the initial stages, where there is intense heat of the body, strong pulse, bright red face and delirium, where the cerebral irritation is marked by intense pain in the head, starting out of sleep crying out, grinding teeth. For simple meningitis, not the tubercular form, when everything is acute and intense; when effusion commences, however, it ceases to be the remedy. Aconite. Meningitis from heat of the sun's rays after long exposure thereto, or cerebral congestions from anger. It is only useful at the onset. Fear is a marked symptom. Veratrum viride. Intense cerebral congestion, rapid pulse, tendency to convulsion, followed by prostration. Elliot considers Veratrum viride in the lower potencies our best remedy in acute meningitis. Coldness of the surface loss of consciousness, dilated pupils, laboured, slow, irregular pulse.

Bryonia 6C to 30C - Suits well cerebral effusions with a benumbed sensorium. The following will be useful indications upon which to prescribe Bryonia. Constant chewing motion with the mouth; when moved screams with pain; child stupid, abdomen distended; tongue white, pains are most sharp and stitching, and the patient drinks greedily; there is a livid flushed face, high temperature, copious sweats. Thus it is seen that Bryonia produces a characteristic image of meningitis and suits especially cases caused by suppressed eruption.

Apis 6C to 30C - Here nervous agitation predominates ; there are shrill cries, stabbing pains ; the child puts its hand to its head and screams. There is an oedematous face, scanty urine, and the patient is thirstless, it suits especially infantile cases and especially the tubercular form due to a developed eruption. Cicuta is useful in the irritative stage when there are general convulsions, twitching in fingers and unconsciousness. It also markedly controls the effusion. The head is spasmodically drawn back with stiff neck. Violent jerks in any part of the body. Strangles on drinking, dilated pupils and staring look.

Helleborus 6C to 30C - Mental torpor marks this drug; a sensorial apathy, there is want of reaction. It corresponds to a later stage of the disease, when effusion has taken place; then symptoms such as wrinkling of one arm and one leg are indicative of Helleborus. There are shooting pains in the head, sudden crying out, screaming, boring head into the pillow. The cries have a most pitiful sound. The patient is cold, pale and pulseless, eyes sunken, face livid. Patient cold, but does not want to be covered.

Zincum Met 6X - This remedy corresponds to the subacute form. Febrile disturbance is absent or slight; there are marked twitching jerkings and hyperaesthesia of all the senses and skin, and tremulousness of the feet. At the beginning there are sharp lancinating pains and great exhaustion of nerve force. Cuprum suits cases marked with violent convulsions, thumbs clenched, loud screaming, face pale with blue lips. No remedy equals it in these conditions, but it is of more use in the later stages.

Covering Nervous Dyspepsia to Strokes

In this section we look at what I think of as mind over body starting with Nervous Dyspepsia and Ulcers leading to Anxiety and Depression. After that we move onto more of the nerve degenerative problems such as Alzheimer's and Parkinson's disease where we try to slow down the damage and repair as much as we can.

Nervous Dyspepsia

Nervous Dyspepsia really means I can worry myself sick, and the bigger your imagination the worse the problem is. This can especially be a problem for children. Here we will only mention digestive herbs with strong actions on the nervous system. Chamomile (have a good look at it in the Herbal) is very important here not only for its obvious reasons and that it is good for children, but because it is high in Calcium and Magnesium which is what the nerves run on, so people with a nervous disposition should always consider supplementation of these especially if they are female because we want to keep the bone density high. Cat Mint (Cat Nip) and Hops are given as herbs below with others to consider being Oats which are soothing to nervous tummies but also a Nervous System Restorative and antispasmodic and Valerian which is our main herbal tranquilizer but is also a Carminative, Antispasmodic and good for anxiety.

Cat Mint

Actions - Carminative, antispasmodic, diaphoretic, sedative, astringent.

This herb is also known as Catnip. Cats and other creatures eat this plant and also give themselves a massage in it. This is an old traditional cold and flu remedy especially for ones with fever. Has an action on the digestive system easing stomach upsets, dyspepsia, wind and colic. Used for diarrhea of the young. Good for the nervous, stressed or restless, helps stomachaches by calming the nerves, used for stress and nervousness. **Dose** - 2 to 4mls of tincture 3 times a day. Good for teas

Hops

Actions - Sedative, hypnotic, bitter, antiseptic, visceral antispasmodic, astringent, nervine.

Famed for its tonic and nervine properties, pain reliever, sleep inducer, antiseptic, tension that leads to restlessness, headache, indigestion, mucous colitis. Good for when digestive problems are caused by worry or nerves. One of the main remedies for IBS. Acts on the central nervous system and calms and eases anxiety. **Doses** - Tincture 1 to 4mls 3 times daily, 1 teaspoon of dried flowers in tea 3 times a day or just before bed. **Caution** - Do not use in depression.

Ulcers Gastric and Duodenal

Nervous Ulcers have been out of fashion now for a long time, but it's interesting to see that some Doctors are now saying high stress and anxiety levels may increase the production of stomach acid which we all know causes the problem. I suspect that the real figure may be around about a third. Stress and worry should always be taken into consideration and investigated for this seems to have an affinity to upsetting the digestive system. The amount of people I know and have treated that can worry themselves sick, especially in the young is so great that it would be foolish to disregard this aspect. I kind of think of it as mind over tummy instead of the letting the brain get on with the job. Being an Iridologist I can see Nerve Rings in the eyes and if there are 3 I can be fairly sure that mind over tummy is at work. Search – Nerve Rings Image. The real name for Nerve Rings is Neurovascular Cramp Rings and they are a very helpful tool. Well now that I have made my point we better get back to the basics. Gastric and Duodenal Ulcers are an erosion through the protective mucous membrane lining allowing the acid to attack unprotected areas causing damage, pain and bleeding. Nearly all ulcers are caused by Helicobacter pylori infection (Ginger) or NSAID Medication because both disrupt normal mucosa defense and healing. Diagnosis is by endoscopy and testing for H. pylori. Ulcers may range in size from several millimeters to several centimeters but it is the depth that they penetrate that is the real problem so for this reason there should be no delay in seeking treatment. See your Doctor and undergo diagnosis so you know exactly where it is and how deep. Helicobacter pylori Infection is present in 50 to 70% of patients with duodenal ulcers and 30 to 50% of patients with gastric ulcers and it has been found that if pylori are eradicated, only 10% of patients have recurrence in peptic ulcer disease, compared with 70% recurrence in patients treated with acid suppression alone.

Gastric Ulcers

These ulcers are in the stomach and often reoccur and turn into a chronic condition so immediate treatment is important. Symptoms can vary depending on the location of the ulcer and some elderly people do not even notice them but for those who do common symptoms can be burning , gnawing, aching pain, soreness or empty hungry feeling in the stomach, a steady pain in a well-defined location that is relieved by milk. To a certain degree the severity of the symptoms depend on the severity of the ulcer. Heart burn is one of the most common signs. In both forms of ulcer there can be bleeding which may be seen in the stool but in gastric ulcers fresh blood may be seen in the vomit. In gastric ulcers, pain occurs 1-2 hours after eating and eating does not seem to relive the pain. People with Gastric Ulcers need to go on a special diet and avoid foods which cause hyperacidity and irritation, such as, spicy foods; creamy and milky foods, such as, milk, cheese, and ice cream. Chocolates and coffee are to be avoided as well. In duodenal ulcers, no special diet is needed. Always remember that milk and dairy foods are proteins and as proteins they need acid for digestion so the milk that just covered and soothed the ulcer soon gives it an acid bath making the condition worse.

Duodenal Ulcers

These ulcers are in the first few centimeters of the small intestines just below the stomach. This is a rather busy area as the pipeline from the pancreas comes in here along with the pipe line from the gallbladder bringing in bile for the digestion of fats. Pain occurs 3 to 4 hours after eating instead of 1 or 2 in gastric ulcers and in this form of ulcer food can relieve the pain. A gastric ulcer has a special diet while duodenal ulcers do not. Other symptoms can be pain that awakens a patient at night, pain that is absent when the patient awakens but appears in mid-morning and pain that is relieved by food, but recurs 2 to 3 hours after a meal. **Herbal Treatment** - Follow the diet your Doctor should have provided and avoid all the irritants or if you are not happy choose one more suitable for your tastes from the internet as there are many there, just keep to the outlines of the Doctors and watch out for spices and excessively hot drink or foods. Cabbage and especially its juice is a very old and effective remedy but in moderation especially if you have a wind problem. The herb we will start with and leave as a background remedy till you are better is Ginger. Ginger is a good digestive remedy more known for treating nausea and motion sickness but a study at the University of Illinois,

Chicago, found that ginger root extracts inhibit the growth of H. pylori the bacteria that has recently been found to be the main culprit in ulcers so ginger will be our back ground remedy taken as a tea made from the fresh root or even in crystallized ginger form. Our main herb will be Meadowsweet the acid balancer, to that we will add Licorice in the extract form (stronger than the tincture) so as to coat and protect the esophagus, stomach, and intestinal lining from stomach acids. In cases of heartburn, licorice also helps repair the stomach's protective mucous lining. A recent study at the Institute of Medical Microbiology and Virology, Kiel, Germany, researchers found that licorice extract produced a potent effect against strains of H. pylori, this is why we are going to use it at the beginning so it can add its actions to ginger. Long term use of Licorice can cause problems so after a week or so we will replace it with Marshmallow. Marshmallow is one of our main Demulcent and soothing herbs that works especially well in the digestive system and is a good replacement for Licorice. The next herb to consider is for bleeding with Cranesbill being our main herb for bleeding ulcers. This herb is a strong astringent which is the action that we use in bleeding ulcers and is a strong anti-inflammatory which will work well with Marshmallows soothing demulcent action. Goldenseal is another specific for ulcers but it can be very hard to find now.

Ginger

Actions - Carminative, anti-inflammatory, vasodilator, stimulant, diaphoretic, anti-emetic.

The therapeutic benefits of ginger are largely due to its volatile oil and oleoresin content. Its antiseptic properties also make it beneficial for gastro-intestinal infections. Aids in fighting colds, colitis, digestive disorders, wind, increases saliva, is excellent for the circulatory system and helps increase stamina and it is also commonly used to help the other herbs in a formula to get into the body. On top of this ginger has a strong antioxidant action that may also help to tone down the inflammatory response. Other uses are for indigestion, nausea, feverish conditions especially when chills are present, travel sickness especially sea sickness, dyspepsia, colic and flatulence.

Dose - Weak tincture 1.5 to 3mls 3 times daily, Ginger tea, crystallized ginger.

Licorice

Actions - Anti bacterial, anti-viral, expectorant, demulcent, anti-inflammatory, adrenal tonic, anti-spasmodic, mild laxative, nutritive. Licorice improves macrophage activity and increases the production of interferon which is antiviral. Licorice extract also has broad spectrum anti-microbial effects along with being an antioxidant protecting the tissues especially those of the liver from free radical damage. The root part is used , licorice is one of our best demulcents especially for sore throats and painful and inflamed airways where it hurts to cough and is also good for gastric ulcers as it coats and soothes them giving them protection and reducing the inflammation, it is also nutritive and slightly laxative, It contains the building blocks of hormones, has a marked effect on the endocrine system and the glands of the body, catarrh, bronchitis, coughs, gastric and peptic ulcers, abdominal colic. Can be used for treating inflammatory and allergic conditions. A recent study at the Institute of Medical Microbiology and Virology, Kiel, Germany, researchers found that licorice extract produced a potent effect against strains of H. pylori which are the main culprits for Peptic Ulcers.

Uses - Treatment of cough, inflamed throat, pneumonia, pleurisy, TB, all catarrhal conditions, gallstones, chronic constipation, arthritis, fatigue, female infertility, pains of colic, stress, easing gastric ulcers, inhibits the herpes simplex virus.

Dose - 1 to 3mls of the tincture 3 times a day.

Caution - Do not use with high blood pressure. Long term use can also raise the blood pressure.

Homoeopathic Remedies for Gastric Ulcers

Arsenic Album 6th to 30C - Burning pains relieved by heat, anxious, restless, weak and chilly with an air of fear and hopelessness. Anxiety or restlessness are often present where this remedy is indicated. Discharge from eyes and nose are watery and acrid causing ulceration in those regions. The mouth is usually dry and the patient is usually thirsty.

Excellent remedy for acid reflux, Foul or sour taste, hot burning sensation in the esophagus and pharynx, eructation of sour, acrid fluid, nausea, retching and vomiting of slimy mucus tingled with blood. Burning pains in abdomen, burns like fire, as if hot coals were applied to the parts. Vomiting of bile, blood, brown black mucus mixed with blood. Severe, burning pain and exhaustion; pain immediately after eating food and a lack of appetite.

Dramatic vomiting and diarrhea often simultaneously indicate its use if the modalities agree. Patients with wheezing respiration and allergic asthmatic conditions can respond well. The skin can be dry, scaly and scruffy. Symptoms are worse for cold and wet better for warmth. Tries to find relief in motion but immediately feels weak with movement. Restless, feels cold, complains of general weakness, discharges burn the skin. Trembling and coldness of extremities with pain in stomach and oppressive anxiety, Irregular and frequent pulse

Mind - Great anguish and restlessness. Fear with despair, anxiety. Changes place continually.

Better - Warmth, open air, relieved by sweat, hot drinks, lying down (but restless).

Worse - Cold air, after midnight eg 1 to 3am. Wet damp weather and near sea shore.

Kali Bichromicum 6th to 30C - Has an affinity for the mucous membranes of the body, tough stringy viscid secretions sometimes forming thick yellow green mucous, sinus infections, suited for fleshy fat light complexioned people, general weakness. Gastric ulcer of the stomach. Pain in small spots, can be covered with the point of finger; appears and disappears suddenly, rapidly shifting. Pain in the epigastric region. Feels as though digestion has stopped. Burning or shooting abdominal pain. Weight in pit of stomach, flatulence, vomiting of stringy, ropy mucus and blood. Loss of appetite. Gastric symptoms are relieved after eating. Vomiting of bright yellow water.

Better - Heat

Worse - Cold, beer, morning, undressing.

Phosphorus 6th to 30C - Irritated and inflamed mucous and serous membranes are the key feature of this remedy. Is a very sudden remedy with suddenness of symptoms. symptoms of acid reflux, heart burn and constant burning in the stomach, regurgitation

of food, Craving for cold food which is vomited as soon as it becomes hot in the stomach, Spitting of blood without nausea is also common in this remedy. Gone, weak feeling in the stomach, burning between the scapulae. A burning, gnawing, circumscribed pain is characteristic. Gums can be ulcerated and bloody. The patient is sensitive to loud and sudden noises (eg thunder fireworks etc). Degenerative processes and bone destruction respond well to Phosphorus. Hepatitis, jaundice, pancreatic disease and nephritis also come into its sphere. Urine may be bloody. A very painful cough is also a symptom. Wounds that perpetually bleed may also be helped. The patient is usually in poor body condition. Rapid loss of flesh and anemia. **Mind** - Low spirits, restless, fearful, fidgety. **Better** - In the dark, lying on the right side, from the cold, sleep. **Worse** - Symptoms are worse for touch, exertion, in the evening and during thunder storm.

Shock

All accidents and emergencies cause a certain degree of emotional shock sometimes very noticeable in children. Shock should always be treated along with any other injuries. Signs of shock can be they look pale, cold and sweaty skin, restless, rapid pulse and there may be shallow and fast breathing. Lay them down and get them comfortable keep them warm and calm and reassure them. Loosen tight clothing. Rescue Remedy is an effective remedy for this condition and can be used for any type of shock physical or emotional. Emotionally it will relieve that uptight feeling or apprehension before a certain event. Rescue Remedy is a mixture of five Bach Flower Remedies and has been used since the late 30s so it has been well proved and is easily found in most health shops and chemists. **Herbal Treatment -** Rescue Remedy - For physical and emotional shock in any circumstances.

Homoeopathic Treatment for Shock

As you would of noticed by now Arnica is our main remedy for shock with Aconite being a very good second remedy if the symptoms match. Don't forget to follow all your normal first aid procedures and keep the patient warm and calm.

Acconite 6C - Severe shock with great fear and restlessness. Fear is so great, person may scream, or say they will die, useful after surgical shock.

Arnica 6C - Reduces shock and hemorrhage and helps relieve the pain.

Anxiety

Anxiety is a general feeling of fear or being worried, usually arising from a cause or perceived threat and can be accompanied by a feeling of unease and may include physical symptoms that may vary in intensity, especially when the imagination gets hold of it and starts playing out all its different scenarios. As adults we all experience anxiety once in a while as this is normal and no doubt when we were young and the world was new we all had a lot more anxiety as we had to experience so many new things as relationships, exams, getting qualifications, licences etc. But the problem begins to get worse if anxiety interferes with your daily life. This can be known as Generalized Anxiety Disorder. Sometimes the anxiety can turn into Panic Attacks. **Symptoms** – Sweating, restless, on edge, got to go to the toilet, muscle tension, trembling, palpitations or fast heartbeat, difficult to breathe or fast breathing, dry mouth or the other extreme, dizziness, insomnia - takes their worries to bed, tics or tremors, desire to escape, stomach upsets, can worry themselves sick, hard to concentrate, headaches and fatigue. Now we have to see if we can find the causes. My belief is most of our anxiety problems are inherited except for those created by the trauma that can be experienced in life, for some of us it was worse when we were children and better when we were adults and for others the other way around. No doubt the children that worried themselves sick at school over tests or bullies grew up and continued on to Anxiety. Mental health problems are one of the hardest paths to walk and to cure. For people like us its best to concentrate on symptoms and what caused or triggered the symptoms and note this all down. If we work this way we can begin to see how deep the problem is and if everything falls to pieces we can give this valuable information to a Professional. **Nutrition** – Exercise, diet and Herbs can all help in the treatment of anxiety. Work with the diet section of the book especially the superfoods. Calcium and Magnesium is what nerves like and the more stressed you are the more you will use. Replace coffee with Chamomile tea as it is probably the Calcium and Magnesium in this tea that relaxes you and calms you instead of getting revved up on the coffee. Next consider the B Vitamins. Nearly every single B vitamin does something to the brain (B6) or the Nervous System but there are problems that we have to be aware of. The first is that the Bs are water soluble so the body can't store them for long and the excess leaves the body in a highly coloured florescent like urine. The second problem is that lots of the Bs work with other Bs, so it is best and cheaper to buy them in B Complex form in a slow release formula and let the body sort out what it wants. Consider taking them daily and after a week or so sit down and have a good think about it and see if you notice a difference. Also check and make sure the blood sugar levels are alright and not going all over the place. **Herbal Treatment** – Start by making friends with Chamomile in the tea form. If you don't like it add a Peppermint tea bag as well to change the taste, you should be able to find them easily in the food store close to the tea and coffee. One advantage of using the tea form is that the small intestines can process it very fast because of the large amount of liquid and send it off to the blood stream to do its work, so always consider this as I am purposely putting herbs that can be used in teas in the Anxiety and Depression sections so you can make your own formulas out of the herbs you find in these two sections that work well for you, so take your time and do it properly and you should end up with a formula that suits you or even a few formulas that you could use for different situations that you have to deal with. (Chamomile and Passionflower are in the Herbal). Schisandra is the main herb we are going to use here which along with being a good anti-anxiety herb is also an adaptogen which means it tries to adapt you to what is happening and to your circumstances. Run this herb for 3 months as it needs time to do its work. Have a read of the herb below. You can add the other herbs mentioned here as and when you think they may be nessesary. Next we move on to Passionflower which is a sedative, relaxant, pain killer and also used for Epilepsy and Anxiety. I think if I had Epilepsy I would always be anxious.

Next consider Lime Flowers which is also in the herbal especially if you have high blood pressure or Cardiovascular problems. We shall end with our two main herbs for this condition which are Valerian and Lemon Balm. Remember to look at Depression which follows as you can use those herbs as well or add them to a formula suited to you. We shall end with Lavender which is good for anxiety and can sometimes prevent depression at the onset and it can be used in tea form as well as in the essential oil form, such as putting the oil in your bath. A lot of the herbs mentioned here can be found in the Essential Oil form, so you should be able to make your own formulas with them as well and a nice long hot bath is a good way to medicate yourself, just don't go to sleep. At the end of the Herbal Section in the book is a section on how to make herbal formulas.

Schisandra

Actions – Adaptogen, immune stimulant, anti-inflammatory, liver and kidney tonic, restorative, nervous system tonic, mild anti-depressant, anti-anxiety and anti-stress, adrenal tonic, antioxidant, astringent, anti-tussive, lung tonic, regulates blood pressure, anti-cholesterol, sedative.

Of great use as a general liver protector that works well in the treatment of hepatitis. It is a liver detoxifier and works to deactivate free radicals that attack liver cells. Being extremely high in powerful antioxidants Schisandra helps to fight against free radical damage, thus lowering inflammatory responses. Can help in the nervous system by increasing the nervous reflex response and can also help in anxiety, depression, neurosis and stress. Promotes vitality and increases memory along with cognitive functions while providing resistance to stress. Is a powerful anti-anxiety herb lowering stress levels and enhancing mental performance. Because of its adaptogenic qualities it specifically reduces both mental and physical stress, exerting a normalising effect on the whole body. Schisandra reduces cortisol levels in the body (the stress hormone) and is effective in controlling changes in serotonin and adrenaline caused by stress. The herb is also considered a lung tonic because it helps the body to better utilize oxygen. Because Schisandra is high in powerful antioxidants it lowers the inflammatory responses, which in turn positively affects, tones and strengthens the immune system along with increasing physical performance and endurance and promotes recovery after surgery. Schisandra has long been used in the traditional medicines of China and Russia for a wide variety of ailments. As far back as 2697 BCE Schisandra was listed in the Yellow Emperor's Study of Inner Medicine, an encyclopedia of healing plants. **Precautions** - Mild side effects may include indigestion, nausea, headaches and skin rash. Schisandra may promote contractions of the uterine muscles and thus should not be used by pregnant women. **Contraindications** - Avoid in fever. **Part Used** - Fruit (berries). **Dose** – Tincture 3 mls up to 3 times daily. Infusions - 1 to 2 tea spoons full to cup of boiling water 3 up to 3 times daily. Can also be found in powder and tablet form.

Valerian
Valeriana officinalis

Actions - Sedative, hypnotic, antispasmodic, carminative, hypotensive, anxiety, emmenagogue, PMS, anti depressive, Nervous System relaxant.

One of the most relaxing nervines available that can be used to safely reduce tension and anxiety and is also a very effective herb for chronic insomnia. Valerian root has been shown to increase GABA (Gamma-aminobutyric acid) levels in the brain which can in turn not only reduce the amount of time taken to fall asleep but can also improve the quality of sleep too.

As an antispasmodic it will give relief to any cramp like and colicky pains and is a good pain reliever in general helping with rheumatic and migraine pains. The essential oil can help in the relief of pain especially if rubbed (diluted) on to the skin for rheumatic conditions or as added to part of a formula. As a pain reliever it is most indicated where that pain is associated with tension such as muscle problems and migraines. Has a powerful muscle relaxing effect on smooth and skeletal muscles and can be helpful in easing menstrual cramps. It can effectively calm the severe uterine muscle contractions experienced by some women during menstruation. GABA also helps to calm anxiety along with valerenic acid and valerenol and also hels in keeping stress levels down and helping in the control of blood pressure. **Precautions** - Not recommended during pregnancy or breast feeding. If it has been taken for a long time it can cause withdrawal symptoms if stopped abruptly. Some individuals will react paradoxically to Valerian and will actually be stimulated by it. Not recommended for those taking barbituates or benzodiazepine medication. **Parts Used** – Root. **Doses** - Tincture 2 to 4mls 3 times daily. 1 to 2 teaspoons full of root in tea 3 times daily or taken when needed.

Lemon Balm
Melissa Officinalis

Actions - Nervous system tonic and relaxant, antispasmodic, carminative, sedative, diaphoretic, frebrifuge, antidepressant, anti-viral, anti-microbial, anti-thyroid, choleretic, mild analgesic, antispasmodic, anti-histamine, hepatic, cardio-tonic and used for hypertension.

Specific use for dyspepsia associated with anxiety or a depressive mood. For digestive relief Lemon Balm is best consumed as a tea taken immediately after meals and also helps the liver and gallbladder. Lemon Balm contains rosmarinic acid an enzyme which increases GABA (gamma amino-butyric acid) in the brain which is one of the inhibitory neurotransmitters used by the brain to prevent over-excitement and attain balance. Increased stimulation of GABA receptors produces a sedative or calming effect which is why it is used as an anti-anxiety herb. This herb combines well with Valerian especially in helping with sleep. Indicated in hyperthyroidism (inhibits TSH (thyroid-stimulating hormone) binding to receptors), anxiety, restlessness, palpitations, headache, and excitability and also is a mild anti-depressant. Can be used for hypertension. Strengthens the brain and its resistance to stress and shock, and lifts the spirits. It has tonic effects on the heart and circulatory system. Can be used topically for gout and internally for rheumatism and neuralgias. Historically Melissa also known as Lemon Balm and was believed to sharpen memory. Lemon balm can also temporarily improve cognitive decline as well as improve the mood for Alzheimer's patients. Another study addressing the use of lemon balm for Alzheimer's concluded that Melissa is one of several plants that may be useful in the prevention and treatment of Alzheimer's disease due to its ability to inhibit acetylcholinesterase and its antioxidant activity. Said to improve cognitive function and reduce agitation in patients. Use this herb for a few months and then take a break for a month and see what happens and make a judgement from that. **Precautions** - Lemon Balm should not be used during pregnancy or lactation. Due to its anti-thyroid action it should not be taken by people with thyroid conditions. Do not take with mental health drugs without advice from a doctor or pharmacist. If you take it when you are sleepy do not drive. **Parts Used** – Aerial. **Dose** – Tincture 2 to 6mls 3 times a day. **Infusion** - 2 to 3 teaspoonful's infused for 10 minutes 3 times daily or when needed.

Homeopathic remedies for Anxiety

Aconitum 30C - A state of fear, anxiety and fright. Emotional and physical mental tensions. For anxiety accompanied by irregular or forceful heartbeat, shortness of breath, or fear of death. **Arsenicum album 30C -** For excessive anxiety that has no clear cause and is accompanied by restlessness, especially after midnight. It also may be used for perfectionists, including children, who worry about everything. Arsenic Album is administered in cases where anxiety accompanies sadness. There is anxiety about health, and about the future. This is attended with intense restlessness. Marked weakness is another prominent symptom of these. Some fears are also there like fear of disease, financial loss, being alone, and of death. It is the best remedy for excessive worriers, particularly for those that obsess about health, can be classified as a perfectionist.

Phosphorus 30C - For an impending sense of doom and anxiety when alone. It also may be used for impressionable adults and children who are easily influenced by the anxiety of others. Restlessness, fidgety, Fearfulness as if something was creeping out of every corner. **Lycopodium 30C** – Afraid to be alone, very sensitive, constant fear of breaking down under stress. For performance and other types of anxiety in those who are insecure, yet hide their low self-esteem with arrogance and bravado. It also may treat children with anxiety accompanied by bedwetting.

Apprehensive.

Argentum nit 30C – Nervous, fears and anxieties. For performance anxiety such as before tests in school-age children with rapid heart rate, feeling of faintness, diarrhoea, or flatulence.

Depression

Here we will deal mainly with simple depression. Depression is a mood disorder that causes persistent feelings of sadness and loss of interest that affects how you feel, think and behave and can lead to a variety of emotional and physical problems. Everyone gets sad and upset but depression lasts longer and interferes with your daily life. Depression can be mild, moderate, or severe. You can have a single episode of depression or depression that comes back or lasts a long time. Major Depression can last for 2 weeks but often it can go on for over 20 weeks. Then we have to look at the causes with a good example being the death of a loved spouse that would really hurt. This example is known as Adjustment Disorder. Another example is Postpartum Disorder of mothers may have depression after giving birth. **Causes -** People with depression may have abnormal levels of brain chemicals called neurotransmitters, including serotonin, dopamine, and norepinephrine. These may contribute to having depression. Also it is beginning to look like depression could have heredity cause as it seems to run in families but more research needs to be done. Nutrition is also another obvious cause so have a good look at the diet section especially think of the B Vitamins, calcium and magnesium. More women than men seem to have depression but this may not be true as women are more open to doctors while men don't tell them much. **Symptoms** – Depression often comes on very slowly so it can be hard to figure out what is happening and sometimes the individual doesn't even know it themselves until a close friend and family member starts pointing out the changes. Look out for continuous low mood or sadness, having low self-esteem, changes in appetite or weight, low sex drive, lack of energy, difficult to fall asleep at night or waking up very early in the morning, irritable and intolerant of others, no motivation or interest in things, avoiding contact with friends and taking part in fewer social activities, neglecting your hobbies and interests, difficulties in your home, work or family life, trouble concentrating. Also look at the Homoeopathic remedies as I have tried to write them as person pictures so as you read them you should be able to imagine that I am describing a person. **Diagnosis** - As depression does not usually go away on its own speak to your doctor so they can run tests to rule out other conditions such as thyroid problems. Most medications for depression take 2 to 4 weeks to start working and may take up to 12 weeks for their full effects to kick in. **Herbal Treatment** – Here we will start with **Oats** as it will do what's needed on the nutrition side. You need to find the least processed Oats (for making porridge) that you can, so go to a Health Shop and buy a big bag of them. Naturopaths will use Oats in the Tincture or Extract form as these take nearly everything out of the Oats that they want. Oats is used for nervous debility and exhaustion associated with depression and is commonly used with Skullcap which is our next herb. **Skullcap** relaxes states of nervous tension while generally helping the whole of the Central Nervous System and for hysterical states. Good for exhausted and depressed conditions. **Vervain** is another good and relaxing nerve tonic that can also ease depression and times of hysteria. Mind and body techniques, such as biofeedback, meditation, and Tai Chi, may help prevent or reduce symptoms of depression. Some types of meditation while not only relaxing, you kind of put a pattern on the brain, imagine that you learnt this meditation months ago before the depression and now that the depression has come on you decide to try it again. In some the brain will jump back into the familiar pattern and give relief to the depression. Think of it as formatting the hard drive.

Withania

Ashwagandha

Actions - Adaptogen, analgesic, anti-tumor, hormone regulator, rejuvinative, anti-inflammatory, sedative, nervous system tonic, immuno-modulator, anti-anemic.

Is used to restore health to the nervous system and eases stress and mental exhaustion as it promotes mental clarity and improves memory and stamina. Good for debility, nervous exhaustion especially due to stress and chronic diseases especially those marked by inflammation. Retards various aspects of the aging process and increases stamina. Promotes mental clarity and improves memory and stamina. Relieves pain by lowering serotonin levels which contribute to the sensitivity of pain receptors in the body. Tonic for the elderly and improves conditions associated with ageing. Promotes recovery after illness and Ashwagandha has many similar benefits to ginseng. It is a powerful antioxidant that is beneficial to the cardiovascular, nervous, endocrine and immune systems but is not as stimulating as ginseng but good for those that have been overstimulated. It has also been shown to be effective against depression. Ashwagandha is one of those rare herbs which is both energising and calming at the same time. It works holistically on the entire body to bring it back to homeostasis and help it to function efficiently. **Precautions** - Pregnant or breastfeeding women should not take Withania. **Constituents** - Withanoloids and alkaoids. **Interactions -** If taken with tranquilizers may cause drowsiness and reduce coordination. **Part used -** Roots and leaves. **Dose** - Tincture – 2 to 3ml taken 3 times per day. Capsules and tablets as dose on the label.

Damiana
Turnera diffusa
Actions - Nerve tonic, antidepressant, laxative, urinary antiseptic, stomachic.
Strengthening remedy for the nervous system, tonic action on hormone system, for anxiety and depression especially with a sexual association, tonic to the male reproductive system for impotence, anxiety and neurosis. Tonic for the aged especially in senile decay. For males it is specially indicated for alleviating problems of achieving and maintaining erections. Damiana also works to relieve stress and anxiety related to fears of inadequate sexual performance. One of the active constituents of this herb is thymol which is a compound that is responsible for Damiana's life enhancing and

stimulating effect on the mind and body. Used for mild to moderate depression, anxiety and nervous exhaustion. Its stimulating and restorative properties make it a valuable herb for anxiety and depression occurring together as can often happen as a result of long term stress. **Contraindications** – Pregnancy. **Parts Used** – Leaves, **Pharmacy:** Infusion: 1 tsp/cup water, TID. Tincture: (1:5, 60%), 1-2 ml TID. **Toxicity -** None reported. **Dose** – Tincture 1 to 2 mls 3 times daily. Infusion 1 teaspoon full to cup of boiling water.

Hypericum
St John's Wort

Medicinal Actions- Anti-inflammatory, astringent, anti-viral, anti-spasmodic, nervine, vulnerary, antibacterial and antidepressant. St John's Wort is perhaps the most studied herb for depression with literally thousands of studies and clinical trials performed to assess its usefulness as an antidepressant. Many studies have found the herb to be equally as effective as traditional antidepressants, but with fewer side effects in mild to moderately depressed patients. This is not meant to be used in major suicidal depression. Taken internally it has a sedative and pain reducing effect, which gives it a place in the treatment of neuralgia, anxiety, tension and general depression. Hyperforin which is a component of Hypericum can inhibit synaptosomal reuptake of serotonin, norepinephrine, and dopamine. It may take 2 to 4 weeks to notice clinical results when taken for depression. Useful in mild to moderate depression, anxiety, neuralgia and myalgia's and generally for pains shooting down nerve pathways. This herb is antiviral both internally and topically. **Contraindications -** Speeds up the elimination of many and can interfere with MAOIs, SSRIs, narcotics and reserpine. Do not use St. John's Wort during pregnancy or lactation. **Caution -** Photosensitivity can occur in susceptible individuals. Fair-skinned individuals should take precautions when exposed to the sun and the elderly should use protective eyewear when exposed also. **Part Used** – Aerial and flowering parts. **Dosage** – Tincture 2 to 4mls three times daily. Infusion – 1 to 2 teaspoonsful of herb infused into a cup of boiling water taken 3 times daily.

Homoeopathic Remedies for Depression

Ignatia 30C – Good for acute cases. Leading remedy for treating depression. Good for cases of acute depression that has just begun. Those who need it remain sad all the time and may have weeping spells. They also isolate themselves and avoid social engagements. They brood all the time lost in deep thought which makes them sad and worried. They may be very irritable. Depression in teenagers. Depression due to grief and worry. Depression that gets triggered by acute grief like the death of a loved one, broken relationships and disappointments in life. Is often best for sensitive people that tend to suppress disappointment or grief. They also do not want to appear vulnerable, defensive, temperamental, or guarded in the eyes of others. Some of the other symptoms may also include insomnia, headaches and abdominal cramps. Not wanting to cry or appear too vulnerable to others, they may seem guarded, defensive and moody. They may also burst out laughing or in to tears, for no apparent reason. Insomnia or excessive sleeping. A feeling of a lump in the throat and heaviness in the chest with frequent sighing or yawning are leading indications of this remedy.

Natrum Mur – 30C - Is used more to treat cases of chronic depression. It is suited to those who are very sensitive, accompanied by sporadic episodes of weeping. They remain absorbed in grief all the time and dwell on the unpleasant memories of the past. They don't like consolation, and it worsens the complaints. They have a tendency to get offended easily. Along with it, they don't have an interest in doing any sort of work. They will often hide inner feelings such as anger, fear of misfortune, grief, or affection. They are also responsible, reserved, guarded, and they seek solitude. Although they also seek sympathy, they can become angry if someone attempts to console them. Anxiety, brooding about past grievances, migraines, back pain, and insomnia can also be experienced when the person is depressed. A craving for salt and tiredness from sun exposure are other indications for this remedy. Other symptoms include migraines, insomnia, back pain, anxiety, and hopelessness.

Aurum Met 30C – For Hopelessness, Worthlessness and Suicidal Thoughts. A remedy for the workaholic with a tendency toward worthlessness, despair, and suicidal thoughts after a failure at work or in their personal life. An effective remedy for depression for patients who are very serious people, strongly focussed on work and achievement, who become depressed if they feel they have failed in some way. Nervous breakdown. Feel that they are worthless and of no value. They assume negative thoughts and the future seems dark to them. They feel that life is a burden, it's useless to live, and they long for death with constant suicidal thoughts. Disgusted of life and thoughts. Profound despondency. Peevish. Rapid and constant questioning without waiting for answers. Oversensitive to noise. Symptoms often worsen at night or during the winter months, but these individuals may find relief from soothing music.

Kali Phos 30C – Depressed after prolonged periods of emotional stress or excitement. It mostly helps people who are over-stressed and have much to worry about. They remain constantly sad, and gloomy. With this, they have negative thoughts in their minds. Those who need it feel mentally and physically exhausted. Mental and physical depression caused by excitement, overwork, worry and insomnia. For a person who feels depression after working too hard, being physically ill, or going through prolonged emotional stress or excitement this remedy can be helpful. Other symptoms that they may present include anxiety attacks, and spells of weeping. Exhausted, nervous and jumpy, they may have difficulty working or concentrating and become discouraged and lose confidence. Headaches from mental effort, sleeplessness, anaemia, sensitivity to the cold, and indigestion.

Sepia 30C - Is an excellent medicine to deal with cases of depression in women during menopause. The most important symptoms present in them are sadness, aversion to seeing family members, and loss of interest in doing any work either mental or physical, even missing out on daily routine activities. They also want to be alone and they may become angry when disturbed. They may feel better after crying but they prefer not to be consoled. There is also indifferent behaviour towards life and family. Such people are constantly lost in worries and are stressed with self-pity. They are very irritable and get offended easily. Sporadic weeping spells seeking consolation, and sympathy. Loss of sexual desire is another major complaint. Other related symptoms include digestion problems and menstrual issues.

Cimicifuga Racemosa 30C - Considered in cases of depression among women that begin after childbirth. Women who need this medicine suffer extreme sadness. They feel that they are enveloped in darkness from which it is difficult to come out. They also feel exhausted by these symptoms. Can be energetic and talkative when feeling well but upset and gloomy when depressed. Other symptoms can be painful menstrual periods and headaches that involve the neck, excessive talking, indifferent behaviour, fear of death, and fear of going mentally insane.

Lachesis 30C – Indicated in cases where delusion is present along with depression such as in cases of psychotic depression. Where people have sadness, feelings of being abandoned, excessive talkativeness, and delusions. Depression can be caused by jealously, suspicion, or repressed feelings, for people who dislike commitment or confinement. Indulges in excessive talking and frequently jumps from one subject to another. A lot of ideas crowd their mind at a given time. When it comes to delusions a person may get suspicious and may feel as if someone may poison or harm them. Other symptoms that appear in them are restlessness, aversion to work, and running away from the world. A person who worries' a lot, very talkative and experiences menopausal depression.

Arsenic Alb 30C – One of the top remedies for depression. Arsenic patients express sadness, restlessness and fear. Anxious, insecure, perfectionistic people who need this remedy may set high standards for themselves and others and become depressed if their expectations are not met. Arsenic Administered in cases where anxiety accompanies sadness. There is anxiety about health and about the future. This is attended with intense restlessness. Good remedy for excessive worriers, particularly for those that obsess about health, can be classified as a perfectionist. They often are depressed when they fail to reach personal high standards. Depression on account of a hidden feeling or guilt. Worry about material security sometimes borders on despair. Marked weakness is another prominent symptom of these. Some fears are also there like fear of disease, financial loss, being alone and of death. The person's symptoms are usually worse in colder weather, and they are also very sensitive to any pain.

Alzheimer's Disease

Alzheimer's disease is the most common form of dementia affecting up to 70% of all people with dementia. The disease damages the brain resulting in impaired memory, thinking and behaviour. The biggest risk factor for having Alzheimer's disease is increasing age with just under a third of people over 85 having dementia. The disease can be either sporadic or genetic. Sporadic can affect adults at any age but usually occurs after age 65 and is the most common form of the disease while the genetic disease is very rare and in people who have the gene flaw the disease may come in their 40's or 50's. The Brain with this ddisease shrinks due to the death of the brain cells. There was also found two types of deposits in the brain. One kind was found outside the brain cells which are known plaques and the other type of deposit was found inside brain cells known as neurofibrillary tangles. The plaques impair synapses so signals cannot pass between brain cells. Tangles kill brain cells by preventing the normal transport of food and energy around the brain cell. Shrinking brains can be diagnosed by a MRI scan. The outer part of the brain is usually the first area affected with short term memory loss being one of the first symptoms. As the disease continues to the deeper parts of the brain the long term memory slowly becomes lost. **Symptoms** - Often begins with lapses in memory and difficulty in finding the right words for everyday objects. Other symptoms can be emotional unpredictability especially when stressed, vagueness in everyday conversation, loss of enthusiasm for previously enjoyed activities sometimes this may not what you think it is. With my mum she didn't like going out to dinner at night any more but the real reason was she was scared of the dark, it just shows that things with this disease are usually not what you think. Memory difficulties especially of recent events, this symptom is one of your main clues as to what is happening. Taking longer to do routine tasks, forgetting well known people or places, inability to process questions and instructions and deterioration of social skills. My mother slipped into what I call survival mode and conman mode. She knew something was wrong but she treasured her independence and could bluff her way through most of the time but after 10 minutes a stranger would start to figure out something was wrong. I could go on for pages but I will just express my sympathy to the careers of these people and for them to take care of themselves. Treatment - They are still working on it. **Herbal Treatment** - Improve blood supply to the brain and nutrition to the brain. For the first we use Ginkgo which opens up the arteries in the neck and in the second think of fish oils, Calcium and Magnesium supplements that are easy to absorb and essential fatty acids with maybe a fish oil supplement especially made for children with Attention Deficient Syndrome which is easy to assimilate and also tastes nicer being the best. Rule out other problems such as low thyroid, allergies, poor digestion etc so as to get a clear idea of what is happening with the Alzheimer's. Sometimes if you are too close to the patient you can't do this and it is better to get someone independent to do it with you and to clearly separate the Alzheimer's from other conditions. This can sometimes make the job easier and allow you to see the real picture. A good example is they may have bad teeth which is what is causing most of the pains and discomfort and also why they are losing weight and bad tempered. Unfortunately this is fairly common especially in those who cannot afford Dental care. It is important to start from a clear picture for your own health as well as there's. Next we start to strengthen the nervous system with nourishing foods such as Qats. The super foods for the Nervous system are Grapes, Millet, Wheat Germ, Brewer's Yeast (all the B vitamins), Oats, Buckwheat and Molasses. Your job is to figure out how to make it palatable. A cup of Peppermint and Chamomile tea with each meal is a pleasant helper for this and maybe a good way of using the Molasses. Next I would use the Herb Bacopa which is more commonly known as Brahmi. This herb improves thinking and memory and as we have hopefully cleared up the picture with our patient we shall put it to work and see if we can get an improvement. This herb has been known to help in Alzheimer's with other symptoms but here we just want to get a simple yes or no. Melissa also known as Lemon Balm is one of the next herbs to consider and used with the Brahami as it may temporarily improve cognitive decline as well as improve the mood for Alzheimer's patients. Another study addressing the use of lemon balm for Alzheimer's Disease, concluded that Melissa officinalis is one of several plants that may be useful in the prevention and treatment of Alzheimer's disease due to its ability to inhibit acetylcholinesterase and its antioxidant activity. Also take a look at the herb Angelica. All that said and done it still remains to be seen. I am mainly thinking of this herb for patients more with anxiety and depression and also because it improves cognitive function and reduces agitation in patients so if these symptoms fit your patient consider this herb. The herb Rosemary has similar Actions and works on the Depression side and has been used for the treatment of Alzheimer's but more based on its complex chemical makeup. (Sage To). For our last herb we are going to use a adaptogen which means this herb will try to adapt you to your condition so you can get the best you can out of yourself. Withania is the name of the herb and it is a rejuvenating nervous system tonic that has served me well for decades. I will stop here as it will take about 3 months to really figure out what the herb has done and to re-evaluate everything. These are extremely hard diseases to get good results from so care, patience and time are needed to see changes. If the patient is happier then you are probably on the right path. Below is the write up on the herb Withania.

Withania

Ashwagandha

Actions - Adaptogen, analgesic, anti-tumor, hormone regulator, pregnancy tonic, rejuvinative, anti-inflammatory, sedative, anti-anemic.

Used to restore health to the nervous system and eases stress and mental exhaustion. Good for debility, nervous exhaustion especially due to stress and chronic diseases especially those marked by inflammation. Retards various aspects of the aging process and increases stamina. Promotes mental clarity and improves memory and stamina. Relieves pain by lowering serotonin levels which contribute to the sensitivity of pain receptors in the body. Tonic for the elderly and improves conditions associated with ageing. Promotes recovery after illness and during convalescence and has great use in various chronic diseases involving inflammation. Can aid bone degeneration, rheumatism, joint pain and neuralgias.

Dose - As on packet.

Lemon Balm

Melissa Officinalis

Actions - Nervous system tonic and relaxant, carminative, sedative, diaphoretic, frebrifuge, antidepressant, anti-viral, anti-microbial, anti-thyroid, choleretic, mild analgesic, antispasmodic, anti-histamine, hepatic, cardiotonic and used for hypertension. Specific use for dyspepsia associated with anxiety or a depressive mood. Indicated in hyperthyroidism (inhibits TSH binding to receptors), anxiety, restlessness, palpitations, headache, and excitability and also is a mild anti-depressant. Can be used for hypertension. It strengthens the brain and its resistance to stress and shock, and lifts the spirits. It has tonic effects on the heart and circulatory system. Can be used topically for gout and internally for rheumatism and neuralgias.

Historically Melissa also known as Lemon Balm was believed to sharpen memory. Lemon balm can also temporarily improve cognitive decline as well as improve the mood for Alzheimer's patients. Another study addressing the use of lemon balm for Alzheimer's concluded that Melissa is one of several plants that may be useful in the prevention and treatment of Alzheimer's disease due to its ability to inhibit acetylcholinesterase and its antioxidant activity. Said to improves cognitive function and reduce agitation in patients. Use this herb for a few months and then take a break for a month and see what happens and make a judgement from that.

Dosage - Can be found in tea, tincture, tablet and essential oil form, all forms will have different dosages so do what the supplier advices. Be careful of using the essential oil form in people with poor livers as essential oils go straight into the blood stream then to the liver.

Homoeopathic Treatment for Alzheimer's

Read all of the below remedies and you will see I am painting a person picture with a personality and their disease. Each remedy shows the picture of a person dealing with their disease which in this case is Alzheimer's disease. If one of these person pictures matches your patient it will have a healing effect or help relieve the condition. Also consider that the person with this disease is still vulnerable to all the other diseases that we all have to deal with such as cold, flu, accidents etc. So if you are using a certain remedy for this condition then it may also work for other conditions. With no escaping end of life conditions it is best to seek a Professional Homoeopath and get them to come to you and see your patient in their own environment and get them to give you 3 or 4 close matching remedies to your patient that also cover a wide variety of diseases. Now you have a number of alternative remedies to use when conditions change and a Homoeopath that knows your patient. A lot of Doctors cross over and become Homoeopaths especially in the UK so if you are lucky you may be able to find one and get two for the price of one.

Nux Vomica 6C to 30C - Patients are often angry, quarrelsome and insensitive to other's feelings; however, they themselves are extremely sensitive to everything and tend to abuse alcohol. Sullen and Faultfinding. Disposition to find fault with everything and every body; extreme sensitiveness to the words and attention of others, inclination to kill his best friends; wants to commit suicide but is too cowardly to do so; very irritable, quarrelsome, vindictive. He or she is very irritable, quarrelsome as well as vindictive. Vertigo with momentary loss of conscious, photophobia worse in morning, cannot sleep after 3am.

Baryta Carb 6C to 30C - Specially indicated in old age especially old men. Loss of memory, mental weakness. Irresolute. Lost confidence in himself. Senile dementia. Confusion. Bashful. Aversion to strangers. Childish grief over trifles. The remedy can help those who are regressing into a fearful behavior, timidity with shyness and lack confidence. There is the loss of memory and some patients may suffer from chronic glandular disorders. Offensive foot sweats.

Conium 6C to 30C - Conium is used to treat the elderly for depression, shyness and fear of being alone. The remedy treats memory loss, as well as relieving the mental confusion and loss of cognitive function that sets in as a result of grief over the loss of a spouse. Conium often helps people regain the ability to concentrate and focus. Great debility in the mornings, weakness of body and mind, vertigo when lying down and when turning in bed, photophobia and excessive eye watering, muscular weaknes in legs, putting feet on chair releives pains.

Parkinson's Disease

Parkinson's disease is a progressive degenerative disorder of the nervous system that affects the Motor Nervous System. This disease occurs in people over 50 and develops gradually, sometimes starting with a tremor in just one hand. While a tremor may be the most well-known sign the disorder also commonly causes stiffness or slowing of movement. Nerve cells lose their ability to synthesise and use dopamine a neurotransmitter in the midbrain. Up to 80 percent or more of these dopamine-producing cells are damaged, dead, or otherwise degenerated. This causes the nerve cells to fire wildly, leaving patients unable to control their movements. Damage to this area of the brain causes muscular rigidity, a pin rolling tremor at rest of the finger and thumb, immobility of the face making it mask like along with a soft monotonous voice with a quaver. The term Parkinsonism is used for a motor syndrome whose main symptoms are tremor at rest, stiffness, slowing of movement and postural instability. Medical Drug treatments aim to increase the levels of dopamine and stimulate the parts of the brain where dopamine works. Treatment can work well but over time things change as the body gets used to the drugs and as these are fairly powerful there are side effects, but research is continuing. Deep Brain Stimulation a little like a pacemaker but giving shocks to the brain has shown good results and hopefully in the future will get better. **Causes** - Mostly unknown but certain gene variations appear to increase the risk of Parkinson's disease so if it's in the family you have a chance of getting it. Environmental triggers such as toxins or injury such as brain tumours, strokes, infections such as encephalitis are other causes. The body uses L-dopa to manufacture dopamine. Dopamine is an extremely important and vital brain neurotransmitter that makes possible the transfer of information from neuron to neuron. Dopamine regulates motor control, sex drive, immune function, growth hormone levels and growth hormone release, and motivational behaviour. This will give you an idea of what may happen in the future and an understanding of my reason in picking the main herb for this condition. **Symptoms** - Signs may vary from person to person and are often mild and go unnoticed. Symptoms begin after 50 and often begin on one side of your body and usually remain worse on that side. A tremor or shaking usually begins in a limb and often in your hand or fingers when it is relaxed and at rest. Muscle stiffness may occur in any part of your body. The stiff muscles can limit your range of motion and cause you pain. Slowed movement comes over time and reduces your ability to move and makes simple tasks difficult. Your steps may become shorter when you walk, there could be difficulty to get out of a chair and you may drag your feet as you try to walk. **Secondary symptoms of the brain -** May be anxiety, depression, insecurity, and stress, confusion, memory loss and dementia is more common in the elderly. **Secondary symptoms of the body** - May be constipation, difficulty swallowing and excessive salivation, diminished sense of smell, loss of dexterity, increased sweating, a slow shuffling gait with small steps on the toes, slowed quieter speech, and monotone voice and urinary frequency and urgency. **Herbal Treatment -** Improve blood supply to the brain and nutrition to the brain. For the first we use Ginkgo which opens up the arteries in the neck and in the second think of fish oils, Calcium and Magnesium supplements that are easy to absorb and essential fatty acids with maybe a fish oil supplement especially made for children with Attention Deficient Syndrome which is easy to assimilate and also tastes nicer. Rule out other problems such as low thyroid, allergies, poor digestion etc so as to get a clear idea of what is happening with the Parkinson's. Sometimes if you are too close to the patient you can't do this and it is better to get someone independent to do it with you and to clearly separate the Parkinson's from the other conditions. This can sometimes make the job easier and allow you to see the real picture. A good example is they may have bad teeth which is what is causing most of the pains and discomfort and also why they are losing weight and bad tempered. It is important to start from a clear picture for your own health as well as theirs. Next we start to strengthen the nervous system with nourishing foods such as Oats. The super foods for the Nervous system are Grapes, Millet, Wheat Germ, Brewer's Yeast (all the B vitamins), Oats, Buckwheat and Molasses. Your job is to figure out how to make it palatable. A cup of Peppermint and Chamomile tea with each meal is a pleasant helper for this and maybe a good way of using the Molasses. Have a good look at the herbs used in Depression, Alzheimer's and Dementia. As Parkinson's is a long term chronic disease you need to use **Adaptogen Herbs**. Adaptogens adapt you to your condition and reduces stress, think of it like hiring a manger to take charge of the situation. The main adaptogens you will be using are Withania, Brahami and Cowhage which is the specific one for this disease which follows. All of these will not work well if there is a poor blood supply to the brain so use Ginkgo with the adaptogen as it opens the arteries in the neck which should increase blood supply to the brain and help get your choice of an adaptogen into the brain. Next herb to consider is Pasion Flower which does a lot of good thing by itself but here we are using it because Passion flower contains two helpful alkaloids harmine and harmaline considered to be effective anti-Parkinson's compounds.

Cowhage

Macuna Pruriens

Actions – Adaptogen, Nerve Tonic, Diuretic, Aphrodisiac, Alterative and Hypotensive.

Mucuna Pruriens is beneficial to brain health as its primary compound levadopa (L-dopa) is a precursor to dopamine, adrenaline and noradrenaline. L-dopa is synthesized in the brain into dopamine which is often used as a treatment in Parkinson's disease. While dopamine is commonly associated with pleasure it actually plays a critical role in muscle control. By raising low dopamine levels this herb can have a positive effect on motivation, attention span and the ability to relax and general mental well-being. As an Adaptogen the herb contains a unique set of phytonutrients that feed the adrenals, balance hormones and significantly reduce stress levels by lowering cortisol. Its libido enhancing effects are thought to be due to the high levels of L-dopa which converts into dopamine in the body. In Brazil the seed has been used internally for Parkinson's disease and other forms of tremors, oedema, impotence, intestinal gas, and worms. It is also considered a diuretic and nerve tonic. Used in Central America as a coffee substitute, whilst in certain parts of Guatemala it is a staple food in tribal diets. Chinese Medicine uses it as an enhancing herb and a prized herb for longevity as well as being a powerful aphrodisiac and adaptogenic herb. **Precautions** - Cowhage can interact with other medications such as those taken for diabetes, antidepressants and antipsychotics. It can also lower blood pressure. **Dosage** - Tincture 2 to 5ml up 3 times daily. Powder form 1 teaspoon up to 3 times daily

Passion Flower

Passiflora incarnata

Actions - Sedative, antispasmodic, anodyne, relaxant, epilepsy, shingles, hypotensive, cardiotonic, vasodilator, diuretic, anti-depressant, nervine relaxant, analgesic.

Passion flower has a depressant effect on the Central Nervous System activity and is also hypotensive. Good for its sedative and soothing properties and to lower blood pressure and to prevent tachycardia. A good herb for insomnia and a very effective herb for nerve pains especially in conditions like shingles. The herbs focus is more on restlessness and irritability, hysteria and anxiety and is soothing to the mentally worried and overworked; it acts on nervousness especially due to unrest, agitation, worry, exhaustion and cerebral excitement. Can be used safely for nervous tension and restlessness, muscle spasm, headaches, irregular sleep patterns, irritability, neuralgias and any condition in which an antispasmodic would be beneficial. Used in the treatment of convulsions, epilepsy, tremors, hypertension, nervous breakdowns, migraines and neuralgias. Passion flower contains two helpful alkaloids harmine and harmaline considered to be effective anti-Parkinson's compounds. **Parts Used -** Flowering tops and leaves. **Precautions** - Do not take Passion Flower if pregnant, breastfeeding or suffering from liver problems. Can interfere with blood thinning and blood pressure medications. Not recommended when driving long distances when tired. **Toxicity -** Mild nerve and muscle irritation with long-term use. **Interactions -**

Additive effect with sleep aids, barbiturates and other CNS depressants. **Doses** - Tincture 1 to 4mls 3 times daily. Weekly max 40 ml. Pause 2 weeks on, 2 days off with long-term dosing. Infusion 1 teaspoon of dried herb in tea 3 times daily.

Homoeopathic Treatment for Parkinsons

Read all of the below remedies and you will see I am painting a person picture with a personality and their disease. Each remedy shows the picture of a person dealing with their disease which in this case is Parkinson's disease. If one of these person pictures matches your patient it will have a healing effect or help relieve the condition. Also consider that the person with this disease is still vulnerable to all the other diseases that we all have to deal with such as cold, flu, accidents etc. So if you are using a certain remedy for this condition then it may also work for other conditions. With no escaping end of life conditions it is best to seek a Professional Homoeopath and get them to come to you and see your patient in their own environment and get them to give you 3 or 4 close matching remedies to your patient that also cover a wide variety of diseases. Now you have a number of alternative remedies to use when conditions change and a Homoeopath that knows your patient. A lot of Doctors cross over and become Homoeopaths especially in the UK so if you are lucky you may be able to find one and get two for the price of one.

Mercurius 6C to 30C - Memory weakened and loss of will power. Slow in answering questions. Weakness of limbs, trembling of extremities especially hands. Pain in joints. Cold and clammy sweat on limbs. Oily perspiration. Weakness with trembling from least exertion. Slow in answering questions. Tremors everywhere in body. All symptoms are aggravated at night, warmth of bed, Damp, cold, rainy weather and during perspiration.

Zincum Metallicum 6C to 30C - Weak memory. Very sensitive to noies. Constant movement of feet. In chronic diseases of the brain, trembling, convulsive twitching and fidgety feet are the guiding symptoms. Violent trembling (twitching) of the whole body especially after emotions. Paralysis of hands and feet. Trembling of hands while writing. Lameness, weakness, trembling and twitching of various muscles.

Gelsemium 6C to 30C - Has a very good effect on nervous disorders. Centers its action on nervous system, causing various degrees of motor paralysis, dizziness, drowsiness, dullness and trembling are the hallmark of this remedy. It is suited to sensitive patients who get excited very easily from sudden fear or emotions. Lack of muscular coordination. Excessive trembling in this remedy, weakness and paralysis of various groups of muscles like eyes, throat, chest, sphincters and extremities. Head remedy for tremors. Mind sluggish and muscular system relaxed. Staggering gait. Loss of power of muscular control. Cramps in muscles of forearm. Excessive trembling and weakness of all limbs. Worse by dampness, excitement, bad news. Better by bending forwards, profuse urination, continued motion and open air.

Vascular Dementia

This is a condition that impairs the blood flow to the brain and one that I see often as a Naturopath. As I am also an Iridologist in my own right I can see this condition immediately when I look into your eyes as it is one of the easiest to see and about the only one in medicine that we agree on. Traditionally through time in medicine it been known as the Arcus Senilis when it's at the top of the eye but Iridologist's usually call them sodium rings. In the coloured part of the eye it looks like a white ring going round just inside the coloured part. In brown eyes it's easy to see but harder in blue, unless it is really thick. This can be seen in three ways, as a full circle, as an arc at the top of the eye or as an arc at the bottom of the eye. I see the arc at the bottom of the eye in heavy smokers and the arc tells me that the main arteries going to the legs are getting blocked which leads you straight away to ask, are you getting cramps in your feet or calves or do your feet feel cold, which is what restricted blood supply does. If the arc is at the top of the eye that tells me the blood flow is being restricted to the brain. Full circles are restricting blood supply to both the head and feet. The immediate thought that rushes into the brain is give Gingko Biloba as its main action is that of a peripheral vasodilator which will open up the arteries' in the neck and thighs and will give us a yes or no answer fairly quickly. **Cause –** Stroke, high blood pressure or something that caused the blood pressure to go extremely high can sometimes cause a blood haemorrhage in the brain. Other causes can be a build-up of plaques inside the arteries, diabetes, and heart failure. Decreased blood supply to the head means that there is a decreased amount of oxygen, which the brain is always hungry for and if the supply remains or gets worse brain function will decrease and lead to permanent injury. **Symptoms** – The most significant symptoms are more the speed of thinking and problem solving abilities rather than the loss of memory. Other symptoms to look out for are unsteady gait, confusion in and deciding what to do next, tiredness and trouble paying attention. Symptoms can be similar to stroke but we will deal with that next. **Treatment** – Depends on cause. If it came on in a long and slow way it would take a while for you to realize there was something wrong. This presentation is the hardening of the arteries type which is getting more dangerous as time goes by as the narrower the artery gets the greater the chance of a clot or a plaque breaking off somewhere else has of blocking off the artery, it's also called old age. Regular check-ups would be a good way to reduce the risk especially if this problem runs in your family. Problems could also be a failing heart along with Angina. So get them to check out the whole Cardiovascular System. **Herbal Treatment -** Gingko Biloba as its main action is that of a peripheral vasodilator which will open up the arteries' in the neck and thighs and will give us a yes or no answer fairly quickly. Next the herb Brahmi will start to repair the damage done to the brain and start to work around and try to rewire what cannot be repaired but may over time be bridged in another way or circuit. Brahmi is an Adaptogen which means it tries to adapt you to your condition so you have to use it for at least 3 months, then stand back and review the situation and see what you think. We will be using Brahmi again in Strokes so as to try to repair the damage, so have a read of that in the Herbal section which will give you more information. I will leave it at that as we continue next with Stroke. After the condition has stabilized consider taking Hawthorn which is below. I will finish here with one of my main hero's which has served me faithfully and helped so many, let me introduce to you Coenzyme

Q-10.

Coenzyme Q-10

A Good Supplement for the Cardiovascular System and those low in oxygen. Coenzyme Q10 Is a vitamin-like substance found throughout the body, but especially in the heart, liver, kidney, and pancreas. It is eaten in small amounts in meats and seafood. It works with the powerhouse or engine of cells known as the mitochondria which is responsible for energy supply. Q-10 rapidly depletes with age. Many people use coenzyme Q-10 for treating heart and blood vessel conditions such as congestive heart failure, angina, and high blood pressure which it seems to reduce a little bit and also seems to have a slight additive affect to blood pressure lowering medication. The Japanese use it a lot for people with heart conditions. Athletes use it to push themselves beyond their normal. My understanding of Q 10 as explained to me by a rep decades ago when it first came out is that it helps the body make energy with less oxygen. Working on that statement I have always used it on patients with conditions such as angina or emphysema or any condition where the body is less oxygenated whether the cause is from poor circulation or poor lung function. I have usually had good results. Q-10 is the only supplement I have been able to experiment with in fairly large numbers of people due to inheriting a massive stock of it just going out of date. I was impressed with the results. In the Chemist I was working in we found out it was really good for hangovers, I could also abort headaches just as they were coming on but with migraines you had to get it exactly at the right time at the very beginning for best results. Everyone with Angina was put on it especially when they had to go out or had lots to do which would require more energy than usual. Some results where exceptional with one elderly Vietnamese gentleman using it just for golf where it increased his range and game with all his friends knowing he was cheating but they could not figure it out. Now I encourage people with energy problems to try Q-10 and see what happens. If they get good results I tell them that this is a good supplement to use when the unexpected happens and if you have to go somewhere or someplace and use more energy than usual such as in an emergency. This helps with confidence and lessens worry. I extensively used it with my father who was in the habit of always pushing himself to far having a failing heart and cancer along with looking after mum with dementia. This basically is the best and fasted working and most helpful supplement I have ever used and for a sarcastic critical sod like me that's saying a lot. Start at a fairly low dose of about 100mg and see what happens. It first came out at about 50mg and I now see them up to and over 500mg. God knows how many the sports cheats take.

Hawthorn
Crataegus oxycantha
Actions - Cardiac tonic, hypotensive, adaptogen, anti-oxidant, coronary vasodilator.
Strengthens the muscles and nerves of the heart, aids in relieving emotional stress, regulates high and low blood pressure, and helps combat arteriosclerosis and heart disease. Strengthens the contractive force of the heart and gently dilates and relaxes the coronary blood vessels. Increases the body's ability to utilize oxygen. This is more of a balancing herb hence the name adaptogen, if the blood pressure is high or low the herb will balance it, if the electrical activity is playing up with rapid or erratic heart beat it will try to balance it which is why it is called an adaptogen. Strengthens and helps to remove plaques from the blood vessels. This is a herb for taking long term. As a long-term treatment it can be used safely in heart failure (cardiac insufficiency) and weakness. Can similarly be used in cases of palpitations, arrhythmia and valvular insufficiency. Will play a role in any treatment of vessel problems including varicose veins or even ulcers. For blood pressure alone add about 500mg daily of magnesium as this can improve the treatment especially if part of the problem is stress. **Heart Failure** - Hawthorn Berries have been extensively studied in relation to congestive heart failure, with findings concurring that symptoms such as shortness of breath and tiredness can be dramatically improved. One study found that 900mg daily of Hawthorn Berry extract was as effective at managing the symptoms of congestive heart failure as its pharmaceutical counterpart. The flavones enhance the function of cardiac enzymes

which can improve the heart's ability to withstand stress. **Interactions -** May help reduce toxicity of cardiac glycosides, hypertensive medications and CNS depressants. **Uses-** As a tonic to the circulatory system and to strengthen the heart. Use for at least 2 months. **Dose -** 2 to 4mls of tincture 3 times a day. Hawthorn Berries - 1 to 2 tea spoons full in cup boiling water up to 3 times a day.

Stroke

A stroke is a medical emergency requiring quick action. Act **F.A.S.T.** which means

Face - Check face, has the mouth dropped on one side.

Arm - Can they lift both arms?

Speech - Is the speech slurred, do they understand?

Time - Is critical to avoid brain damage, call ambulance.

A stroke happens when the supply of blood to the brain is suddenly interrupted by a clot or a bleed from a burst vessel, the problem is we won't know which till latter. Some strokes are fatal while others cause permanent or temporary disability. Facial weakness, arm weakness and difficulty with speech are the most common symptoms or signs of stroke, other signs can be weakness, numbness or paralysis of the face, arm or leg on either or both sides of the body, dizziness, loss of balance or an unexplained fall, loss of vision, sudden blurring or decreased vision in one or both eyes, a headache, usually severe with abrupt onset or unexplained change in the pattern of headaches and difficulty swallowing. Treatment with Natural Remedies with the exception of Homoeopathy can only really begin after the emergency is over and the cause is known with the patient stabilized. Let the Paramedics know if you have given a Homoeopathic remedy as it could mask some symptoms. **Herbal Treatment -** Start work on hardening of the arteries and getting blood pressure under control so as to reduce risk of a reoccurrence and stabilize the condition. First we will concentrate on recovery after the stroke. Generally I use Ginkgo which opens the arteries in the neck and allows me to target the Brahmi to the head which is my main herb. Generally once a nerve is dead that's it, though there is hope from the new research being done on drugs and stem cells. After a stroke there is sometimes seen after a period of time and a lot of effort on the patients part a rewiring of nerves around the damaged or dead area, this is what we are trying to do with the Brahmi. Some of the new technology which uses games requiring movement has found that it takes 10,000 movements to see the first changes; I am hoping Brahmi makes that less. The Ginkgo is helping by increasing blood flow along with the nutrients and oxygen it carries but now comes the hard part which is getting the areas affected to work again. I try to use Brahmi as follows, for example let's say the left hand is partially paralysed (Shizandra for nerve repair) strap the good arm to the side or sit on the hand so the arm cannot be used and concentrate on using the damaged arm. You are looking at months of doing this as nerves don't grow over night but it has been known to get results and I have had a lot of success with Shizandra. Try to incorporate this idea into your physiotherapy recovery program. Shizandra is very useful for mini strokes as they usually do not cause as much damage as the severe ones do especially in the arms and legs. I have found this herb very useful in the arms where the nerves have been damaged causing loss of strength, shooting pains and sometimes suddenly dropping things especially if they have a bit of weight in them. A good way to start in sorting this out is to go to a Physiotherapist and get them to test your reflexes in pairs. For example, they test the reflex in the biceps of the arm, the right one does a big twitch but the left one only does a little twitch, this shows you the left arm is working on less nerve power. Time to put Shizandra to work for 3 months along with exercising the arm, then back for a reflex check. These damaged nerves can also be sending shooting pains and aggravating other parts of the arm.

Brahmi

Bacopa

Actions - Anti-inflammatory, Anti stress, Anti-oxidant.

Bacopa Monniera is one of Ayurveda's most investigated and documented herbs which acts as a brain and nervous system tonic. Often prescribed for epilepsy, psychiatric disorders such as a mental breakdown, dementia, Alzheimer's, neuralgia, poor concentration and memory. The herb is used for memory loss, poor concentration,

Alzheimer's disease, Attention Deficit Disorder, nervous deficit due to an injury, stroke or transient ischemic attack, nervous breakdown or exhaustion and to improve circulation, strengthen capillaries and stimulate hair, skin and nail growth. Brahmi possess no known side effects or toxicity at normal doses. **Dose** - I generally use this with Ginkgo which opens the arteries in the neck and allows me to target the Brahmi to the head. If you look hard enough you should be able to find these two already mixed together usually at about the same strength. Take as dosage on the bottle.

Schisandra

Actions – Adaptogen, immune stimulant, anti-inflammatory, liver and kidney tonic, restorative, nervous system tonic, mild anti-depressant, anti-anxiety and anti-stress, adrenal tonic, antioxidant, astringent, anti-tussive, lung tonic, regulates blood pressure, anti-cholesterol, sedative. Of great use as a general liver protector that works well in the treatment of hepatitis. It is a liver detoxifier and works to deactivate free radicals that attack liver cells. Being extremely high in powerful antioxidants Schisandra helps to fight against free radical damage, thus lowering inflammatory responses. Can help in the nervous system by increasing the nervous reflex response and can also help in anxiety, depression, neurosis and stress. Promotes vitality and increases memory along with cognitive functions while providing resistance to stress. Is a powerful anti-anxiety herb lowering stress levels and enhancing mental performance. Because of its adaptogenic qualities it specifically reduces both mental and physical stress, exerting a normalising effect on the whole body. Schisandra reduces cortisol levels in the body (the stress hormone) and is effective in controlling changes in serotonin and adrenaline caused by stress. The herb is also considered a lung tonic because it helps the body to better utilize oxygen. Because Schisandra is high in powerful antioxidants it lowers the inflammatory responses, which in turn positively affects, tones and strengthens the immune system along with increasing physical performance and endurance and promotes recovery after surgery. Schisandra has long been used in the traditional medicines of China and Russia for a wide variety of ailments. As far back as 2697 BCE

Schisandra was listed in the Yellow Emperor's Study of Inner Medicine, an encyclopedia of healing plants. **Precautions** - Mild side effects may include indigestion, nausea, headaches and skin rash. Schisandra may promote contractions of the uterine muscles and thus should not be used by pregnant women. **Contraindications -** Avoid in fever. **Part Used -** Fruit (berries). **Dose –** Tincture 3 mls up to 3 times daily. Infusions - 1 to 2 tea spoons full to cup of boiling water 3 up to 3 times daily. Can also be found in powder and tablet form.

Homoeopathic Treatment for Stroke

This is a straight lift from Doctor W A Dewey's book now copyright expired. Doctor Dewey treated this condition in the 1920s and 30s so I thought it best to keep my mouth shut and give you the words of a true Professional in action and it gives you a chance to see true Homoeopathy in action by a man on the spot who most likely wrote this as a personal reference to use during his work.

Opium 3rd to 30th and 200C - The remedy undoubtedly most similar to the general symptoms of stroke is opium. It has a dark red flushed face and the darker the better the indication. It has rattling strenuous breathing and unconsciousness, with sometimes a tetanic rigidity of the body and paralysis. The pulse is exceedingly slow and full, and there is drooping of the lower jaw; stroke in drunkards suggests this remedy, Nux vomica or Sepia. Marked venous congestion is a more valuable symptom than profoundness of stupor. Ferrum phosphoricum. Dr. E. G. Jones uses this remedy in the 3x trituration in hot water when called during an apoplectic seizure, stating that it will usually restore the patient to consciousness in a short time and also control the haemorrhage. Here Aconite may be a better remedy if the mental anxiety is very prominent. Kali muriaticum. The same author uses this remedy to absorb the exudate and believes that many lives may be saved by its use.

Arnica 3rd to 30C - Is the remedy where there is soreness and aching all over the body, paralysis, especially of left side, full, strong pulse and stertorous breathing. Bed sores form rapidly. It is a remedy to prevent threatened stroke. Often attacks of stroke can be prevented by restoring the circulation to its equilibrium by means of such remedies as Aconite, Belladonna, Glonoine and Arnica. Bayes attributes many cases of stroke in old people to the habit of taking medicines to keep their bowels open. This should lead us to treat carefully the constipation, and here opium may perform a double action. Stroke due to external violence calls for Arnica. It should be administered after acute symptoms have subsided to promote absorption of the clot, and here the 30th potency has acted very promptly. Dr. Wm. Morris Butler believes that we have in Arnica 30 a sheet anchor for dissolving blood clots in our own hands it has worked most favourably in a number of cases.

Belladonna 3rd to 30C - Here we have red face, loss of consciousness, convulsive symptoms, dilated pupils, difficult deglutition, involuntary emission of urine, coma and sopor. Hyoscyamus is similar; patients fall suddenly with a shriek and pass into a condition of sopor, with involuntary faeces. Glonoine is indicated buy high arterial tension and co-existing kidney disease. Severe and sudden congestion.

Degenerative Nerve and Muscle Conditions

These can include Peripheral Neuropathy, Myasthenia Gravis and a few more. Treatment of these degenerative conditions of the nervous system will depend on the cause of each individual situation. **Symptoms** - Symptoms of neuromuscular disease vary according to the condition and may be mild, moderate or life threatening. Some of these symptoms may be muscular weakness, muscle wastage, muscular cramps, muscle stiffness which later causes joint or skeletal deformities, muscle pain, breathing difficulties such as intercostal rheumatism or swallowing difficulties which could be related to dementia. **Causes May Be** - Genetic mutation, viral infection, a autoimmune disorder, a hormonal disorder, a metabolic disorder, a dietary deficiency, drugs and or poisons or toxins especially if they are a farmer. Some of the major diseases which affect the neuromuscular system are classified into four main groups. **Motor Neurone Diseases** - where for unknown or genetic reasons the lower and sometimes also the upper motor neurons gradually die. **Neuropathies (nerve diseases)** – the peripheral nervous system is affected. Some of the different diseases of the peripheral nerves include the genetic disease Charcot-Marie-Tooth disease, diabetes especially in the aged who have had it awhile and autoimmune diseases such as chronic inflammatory demyelinating neuropathy (CIDP). **Neuromuscular junction disorders** – in these diseases the transmission of the signal to move a muscle is blocked as it tries to bridge the gap between the nerve and muscle. Myasthenia gravis is the most common of these diseases which is an autoimmune disease where the immune system produces antibodies that attach themselves to the neuromuscular junction and prevent transmission of the nerve impulse to the muscle. **Myopathies** (muscle diseases) including muscular dystrophies – many different types of muscular dystrophy (muscle wastage) are caused by various genetic mutations such as Becker muscular dystrophy and Duchenne muscular dystrophy. Other diseases of the muscles can be caused as a rare side effect of medications such as statins, autoimmune diseases such as polymyositis or polymyalgia rheumatica or hormonal disorders such as hypothyroidism. **Herbal Treatment -** First start with the disease and cause. Strengthen the immune system in auto immune or allergy based diseases affecting the nervous system.

Immunity

Chronic - Echinacea, Hypericum, Phyllanthus. Astragalus, Siberian Ginseng.

Acute - Propolis, Boneset, Pleurisy Root, Picrorrhiza, Hypericum, Echinacea.

Allergies - Albizzia, Feverfew, Baical Skullca , Chamomile, Garlic.

Liver / Toxicity - Licorice, Bupleurum, St Marys Thistle, Dandelion Root, Rehmania, salvia.

 Liver restoratives may be very helpful in decreasing the effects of toxicity eg from alcohol or chemical exposure.

Nervous restoratives

Oats, Gotu Kola, Damiana, Schisandra, Bacopa, Vervain, Rosemary, Skullcap and Withania.

Herbs are very effective with the diet in helping stabilise blood sugar, promote breakdown and assimilation of nutrients and to relieve food intolerances and improve nutritional balances. Some of the nervines are known to have a direct effect on nerve tissue and may improve nerve impulse transmission.

Anti-Inflammatory - Guaiacum, Devils Claw, Black Cohosh, Willow Bark, Licorice.

Antispasmodics - Skullcap, Black Haw, Valerian, Passion Flower, Wild Yam and Cramp bark.

Antispasmodics help ease spasms and jerky uncoordinated movements while other nervines nourish and strengthen the nervous system.

Anti- inflammatorys may also be helpful in treating underlying causes of the nerve and muscle diseases.

Circulatory Stimulants - Ginger, Cayenne, Prickly Ash, Bayberry

Circulatory stimulants in promote the blood flow and nutrition to the nerve centres and helping relieve numbness etc. A good herb to think of here is Ginkgo as this is a peripheral vaso dilator which increases blood supply to arms, legs and the head which in turn increases oxygen and nutrition level to the affected area. This herb will also help target you chosen herb to the area you want.

Covering Encephalitis to Chronic Fatigue

Encephalitis can turn out to be a number of different diseases and in some cases turn into Meningitis which we have already looked at but it's scary where what begins as a headache can take you to. My first experiences with people who had this condition were in helping them with Chronic Fatigue. Most of them were victims of Mosquito Diseases mainly Ross River Fever. These conditions are becoming common now due to climate change which is why I chose Murray Valley Encephalitis for the disease write up as its treatment is similar to Japanese Encephalitis and Dengue Fever which are all present and on the march where I live. Just knowing what to do in a fever can save lives especially when it comes on fast and you don't know what it is, so take a good look at the fever section and if you are worried just call an Ambulance.

Encephalitis

Encephalitis is an infection of the brain more commonly caused by a virus. Old and other causes are HIV, poliovirus, rabies and viruses associated with childhood diseases such as measles, mumps, and rubella. One of the main causes of viral encephalitis is the Herpes viruses, especially the herpes simplex virus (cold sores, shingles) for which there is good medication for treatment. The Herpes Simplex Viruses are responsible for about 10% of encephalitis cases in the USA. The next main cause is Arboviruses which means they are spread to people by the bites of infected insects such as mosquitoes and ticks. Encephalitis can start with a headache and also cause Meningitis which is why I went into great detail in the Headache Section as you can never really know where a headache can take you. In very rare cases, encephalitis can also be caused by bacterial infection, protozoa, or as a complication from other infectious diseases. **Symptoms** - Appear within several days to weeks of exposure to the virus. First signs can be flu like symptoms. Most develop headache and sensitivity to bright light along with weakness, nausea and tiredness. If the case starts to become severe a high fever will develop followed by a severe headache along with a stiff neck and back. There can be vomiting, muscle weakness and drowsiness with confusion. There can be seizures especially if the temperature gets too high. Up to 50% of people with encephalitis may have seizures. Severe cases of encephalitis can have swelling of the brain caused by excess fluid or bleeding within the brain or nerve damage, but this is fairly rare now but shows that prompt intervention is very important. If in doubt just ring for an ambulance as the operators are well trained now and let them sort it out. **Prevention** – Insect repellent and fly or insect screens especially around the bed. Also do not travel to areas where viral encephalitis is common especially if you have a weakened immune system or are unwell or run down. For children make sure they are vaccinated for measles, mumps, and rubella (MMR Vaccine). **Treatment** – Is usually with anti-viral medication and monitoring the patient's condition especially during the fever. **Prognosis** - Full recovery can take weeks or months. Serious cases may have complications ranging from fatigue and trouble concentrating to tremors and personality changes. **Herbal Treatment** - Here we start after the main crisis and fever is over and we are sure of survival for the patient. The first herb is Echinacea which is going to start to rebuild the immune system by getting the white blood cells back to where they should be. Next is Garlic Oil in capsules which should be easy to find. Garlic is antibacterial and antiviral and as we are using this in the oil form it will cross over into the blood stream very fast and to prove it you will have garlic breath as some of it escapes via the lungs. The brain and head has a very big blood supply which is now carrying a strong antiviral which is going to hopefully mop up the remaining viruses. After this we start Astragalus whose main job is to prevent Chronic Fatigue and take out any viruses that are left and restore the immune system back to what it should be. As an adaptogen it will work like a tonic and tone up the body. Run for 3 months which is the blood cycle. (Red blood cells are replaced every 3 months which is known as the blood cycle).

Astragalus

Astragalus membranaceus

Actions - Immuno-modulator, anti-viral, adaptogen, hypotensive, immune stimulant, adrenal tonic, diuretic, vasodilator, cardiotonic, antioxidant, hepatoprotective, hypoglycemic.

This herb is usually used in chronic diseases as a preventative or in cases of fatigue especially in chronic diseases. Stimulates the natural production of interferon and intensifies the white cell destruction of germs. A good tonic for strengthening the resistance to disease. Is very useful for chronic debility and fatigue by restoring the immune function. Use as a lung tonic to help expel toxins and pus in flu's, colds and sinusitis. Increases stamina and can accelerate wound healing, can help to replenish bone marrow. Strengthens the digestive system and aids adrenal gland function. This herb is used for cancer especially if the patient has had chemotherapy and helps aid them in their recovery. Thought to control body fluids such as excessive sweating, night sweats and relieve fluid retention. Astragalus has powerful anti-aging properties slowing the aging process at a cellular level. Astragaloside IV a saponin has shown benefits in reversing cell damage and in activating telomerase, this addresses telomere shortening and slows down cellular aging. This is very important, I will try to explain. Inside every cell of your body is a Telomere, a good way to think about it is as an hour glass. Every time a cell divides it breaks a little piece of the telomere off which is a bit of sand flowing through the hour glass, when the last piece of the telomere is gone that is the last time the cell can divide, this is how we age. Now I will explain why Antioxidants are so important. Imagine a nasty little free radical with a baseball bat which has just smashed into one of your cells and is wandering round inside and then comes across the telomere and says I will fix you and smashes the telomere right at the bottom and leaves only a little stump left. That's it for the cell, life has been cut short. Astragalus root is most effective when taken long term, providing many benefits that can contribute to a longer, healthier life. Good to use for chronic fatigue syndrome (CFS) and fibromyalgia. Has cardio protective affects helping to prevent plaque buildups in the arteries and narrowing of the blood vessel walls, by protecting the inner wall of the vessel. It has also been shown to reduce blood pressure and lower triglycerides. **Immune Boosting -** Is an immune stimulant that it is known to increase the count of white blood cells and stimulate the production of antibodies, this builds up bodily resistance to viruses and bacteria. Many clinical studies have shown it boosts the immune system and encourages an increase in immune T-cells, natural killer cells, macrophages and immunoglobulin activity, production, and function. Astragalus appears to trigger immune cells from a resting state into heightened activity. The natural killer cells of the immune system also seem to be markedly enhanced to fight intruders five to six times higher than normal. **Cautions -** Should not be used in acute infections or fevers. Use with care for those with very low blood pressure. Women who are pregnant or breastfeeding should not use Astragalus. May counteract anti-diabetic agents, and potentiate effects of diuretics.

People with autoimmune diseases should consult their healthcare professional before using Astragalus because of its ability to stimulate the immune system. **Part used -** Root **Dose -** 500 to a 1000mg per day or up to 20 drops of tincture twice daily.

Garlic

Allium sativum

Actions - Immune stimulant, anti-bacterial, anti-viral, anti-fungal, anti-septic, anti-oxidant, diaphoretic, cholagogue, hypotensive, anti-spasmodic, vermifuge and many more.

The plant is rich in volatile oil and Sulphur and because of its remarkable penetrating, disinfecting and mucous expelling powers garlic is a valuable basic remedy for the treatment of all ailments in which the cleansing of the blood stream and expulsion of mucous accumulations is required. Garlic is one of our main herbs used to prevent and treat respiratory infections. Anyone who has had garlic breath has experienced this herb's aromatic compounds being excreted through their lungs which is why garlic's active ingredients can be so effective for respiratory complaints. Garlic is extremely effective in dissolving and cleansing cholesterol from the blood stream, it stimulates the digestive tract, kills worms, parasites and harmful bacteria, normalizes blood pressure and reduces fever, gas and cramps. I use Garlic in oil form (Garlic Oil Capsules) for respiratory infections as the oil goes into the blood stream fast and a lot of it exits via the lungs hence the garlic breath. **Uses -** All infections, coughs, colds, flu, bronchitis, all fevers, pulmonary conditions, gastric and skin complaints, rheumatism, all worms and ringworm, ticks and lice. Acts on Bacteria, Viruses and Internal Parasites. **Dose –** 3000mg Garlic Oil tabs are the best way to go as it gets into the blood fast. For those who cannot tolerate the breath use Kyloc the Japanese aged form as this is odorless.

Fever

Normal body temperature is considered to be 98.4 degrees (37C) but can range between 96 to 99 degrees (35.6 to 37.2C). Onset of a fever can be gradual or sudden and the temperature can remain fairly normal during the day time but rise dramatically at night. Fever is one of the body's main defense mechanisms as the extra heat speeds up the chemical reactions in the body and hinders the germs as they do not like excessive heat, so fever is the body's way of taking the battle to the invader. As the temperature raises so will the pulse and respiration and as the temperature goes down so will they. In herbal medicine we support the fever because it has a job to do, the idea is to keep the fever out of the danger areas, in other words not too high but not too low. Herbalists treat fevers with herbs that are called Diaphoretics. Diaphoretics are herbs that cause the body to sweat, they mimic the action of fevers and rid the body of toxins and can reduce the fever in a short time. We use the Actions of Febrifuges when the body temperature gets into the danger areas and needs to be brought down a good example would be Dengue Fever. Take the temperature frequently so you know which way it is going. Drink plenty of fluids. If the temperature is very high one should begin sponging, this should be done with just warm water and should not be overdone. Start sponging only the forehead and face and observe the effect on the temp. If the temp drops below 102 the sponging can be stopped. If more extensive sponging is required the extremities and the torso can be moistened. Do not attempt to drop the temp back to normal as this will merely suppress the fever and likely chill the patient.

Normal Temp Is	37 C	98.6 F
Oral Ranges	36 to 37.5	96.8 to 99.5
Rectally	0.5 higher	1 F higher
Axillary	0.5 lower	1 F lower

Because of the differences the number is followed by the method taken.
1. Low grade fever - 37.5 to 38.2 C or 99.5 to 101 F
2. High grade fever - 38.2 C above this or 101 F and above.
Fevers can rise dramatically at night. As the temperature rises so will the pulse and breathing rate with the amount of urine passed reduced and concentrated due to the sweating. Other symptoms such as lassitude, feelings of hot and cold, shivering and aches and pains in the back and limbs are common. If the temp rises above 103 (39.4

C) delirium may occur which may lead to convulsions and finally coma if no attempt is made to reduce the temperature. Convulsions are fairly common in children between the ages of 1 and 3 but are rare after the age of 5. **Treatment** - Keep fever out of the danger areas, not to high not to low, give diaphoretics to reduce heat and cause sweating for the removal of toxins e.g. Peppermint and Ginger tea hot and at frequent intervals to promote sweating. Give hot teas at frequent intervals to promote perspiration. After the temperature has returned to normal the teas may be taken cold for their tonic properties. The teas can be taken every one or two hours hot in about 60mls doses until perspiration has taken place. A lot of this depends on the patient if they want a bit more give it to them. Patients with dry fevers i.e. no sweating usually feels agitated, restless and distressed and may be in some danger. High dry fevers should be treated with herbs that relax and **Moisten** e.g. Yarrow, Chamomile, Elder, *Boneset and Pleurisy root.*

For **Sluggish Fever** give stimulants - *Ginger, Cayenne, Horse Radish.*

Herbal Treatment

Peppermint tea - diaphoretic, cooling.

Ginger - diaphoretic, circulatory stimulant, these two actions make ginger good for a fever that has chills.

Chamomile has a good all round action but the herbs above are the main ones for fever though you could mix some of them together.

Herbal Actions for Fevers

Diaphoretics - These herbs are used for fevers and aid the skin in the elimination of toxins and promote perspiration. - Angelica, Boneset, Catnip, Cayenne, Elder Flower, Ginger, Hyssop, Lemongrass, Lemon balm, Penny Royal, Peppermint, Pleurisy Root, Yarrow.

Febrifuge - Helps the body to bring down fevers.

Herbs - Angelica, Boneset ,Cayenne, Elder Flowers, Hyssop, Marigold, Penny Royal, Peppermint, Plantain, Raspberry, Sage, Thyme, Vervain.

Rehydration Formulas

Dehydration and severe diarrheal diseases particularly in epidemics are massive killers (Cholera) in the third world especially among children. The death rate is dramatically reduced now due to the use of Oral Rehydration Solution (ORS) packed into millions of sachet and sent around the world by the World Health Organization. Many diseases can dehydrate you not only from diarrhea but also from the fever and vomiting alone, so great care must always be paid to dehydration in any disease. In the western world hospitals they don't use ORS but use the IV drips instead but if there is a massive pandemic then we all have to look after ourselves so let's get used to the idea of making and using Oral Rehydration Solutions now and of always keeping an eye open for the possibility of Dehydration in any condition. Remember when you make your own ORS that ingesting plain water does not help restore the salt content of the body. But ingesting water with too much salt will draw fluids from the body, and make the dehydration worse. Sugar is also added to the ORS solutions for two reasons. First because sugar helps with the transport of fluids across the cellular membranes in the bowel and second because sugar also provides needed calories to keep the strength up but as with salt too much sugar can be detrimental, it can promote diarrhea and make the loss of fluids worse. **Symptoms of dehydration** can be weakness, headache and fainting, dryness of the mouth, decreased saliva, lack or very decreased urine that is dark in color and highly concentrated, sunken eyes, loss of the elasticity of the skin, low blood pressure especially upon sitting up or rising from the sitting to the standing position and a fast pulse when laying or sitting up.

Formulas

1. The simplest formula is 3 Tablespoons of sugar and 1 teaspoon of salt dissolved in 1 quart of potable water.

2. An alternative simple formula is 8 teaspoons of sugar and 1 teaspoon of salt dissolved in 1 quart of potable water. This basic formula has been used effectively for more than 40 years by WHO.

3. A slightly more complicated formula may be used to replace lost potassium, and to help control diarrhea. This formula is from Dr. Steven J. Greenwald and is designed specifically to
help people who were being threatened with extreme diarrhea.

ORAL REHYDRATION FLUID FORMULA

1/4 teaspoon Salt (common table salt - sodium chloride)
1/4 teaspoon Salt Substitute or "Lite Salt" (potassium chloride)
1/4 teaspoon Baking Soda
2 ½ tablespoons Sugar
Combine these ingredients and dissolve them in 1000 ml (1 liter) of sterile water.
Chemists and Drug Stores should be able to help with any problem here.

Murray Valley Encephalitis

Murray Valley encephalitis is a mosquito-borne disease caused by the Murray Valley Encephalitis virus. It is also known as Australian Encephalitis. The virus is spread by the bite of an infected mosquito (usually *Culex annulirostris* also known as the "common banded" mosquito). Not all of these mosquitoes carry the virus, and only about 1 person in a 1000 who get bitten by infected mosquitoes will become unwell. The virus is thought to be mainly carried by water birds. Mosquitoes become infected by biting birds or other animals that carry the virus. Spread to south eastern Australia is thought to occur with water bird migration that follows unusually wet conditions in inland Australia. **Disease Process** - Murray Valley encephalitis virus is a flavivirus. It has the capacity to cause severe human disease, with encephalitis being the most notable clinical feature. It can commonly infect humans without producing apparent disease (subclinical infection), or it may cause a comparatively mild disease with features such as fever, headache, nausea and vomiting. In a small percentage of people infected, mild disease may be the beginning of disease progression and involvement of the central nervous system, causing meningitis, or in the worst scenario, encephalitis of variable severity. Signs of brain dysfunction, such as drowsiness, confusion, fits, weakness, or ataxia, indicate the onset of encephalitis. **Diagnosis** - MVE is diagnosed when a blood test or test of the spinal fluid shows evidence of the virus (through nucleic acid testing or a rise in antibodies). A diagnosis of MVE disease should be considered in any patient who presents with encephalitis or central nervous system symptoms and who has been in the MVE endemic area within the incubation period of the disease, especially in the period between November and July. **Prevention -** There is no specific treatment or vaccine available for MVE. The only protection is to avoid being bitten by mosquitoes. This is particularly important to travelers and visitors to areas where the disease might be active. **Symptoms** - The disease takes about 5 to 15 days (normally 7 to 12 days) between getting bitten and becoming sick. The majority of people infected will have no symptoms. Of those who do, symptoms can include high fever, severe headache, seizures or fits (especially in young children), tremors, neck stiffness, lethargy, irritability, drowsiness, vomiting, nausea, diarrhea, dizziness, confusion and coma in severe cases. When encephalitis develops, brain dysfunction may be experienced after a few days with lethargy, irritability, drowsiness, confusion, convulsions and fits; neck stiffness can be expected, and both coma and death may ensue. **Prognosis** - People most at risk are babies, young children and newcomers to the region. The disease is fatal in about 20 per cent of those who become sick, and a further 25 per cent can develop major neurological complications. About 40 per cent of cases will make a complete recovery. **Treatment** - Patients with MVE will usually require extensive support sometimes in an intensive care unit in hospital.

There is no specific treatment for MVE. **Herbal Treatment -** As usual you should have started off with our main Disease Fighting Herbs (Echinacea, Garlic and high doses of Vitamin C) which have hopefully made this a much milder version of the disease. For this disease you really don't want to get a bad case. Treat the symptoms as they come using the Actions needed. For the fever we are going to use Boneset as it is good for the aches and pains of flus and fevers. This herb works by inducing sweating so toxins are eliminated through the skin and fever leaves the body. Look at the Fever and Rehydration section a few pages back and take from it what you need. If the temperature is getting to high just ring an ambulance as mentioned before and maybe start sponging down the legs arms and face. To this think of adding St John's Wort as this is a Nervine

Antiviral (especially for the Herpes Virus) that we can use for any virus attacking the nervous system. Instead of using Licorice to force the formula into the body use Ginkgo Biloba as this opens the arteries in the neck and is good for getting the herbs you want into the brain as it increases the blood flow to the head and also has a strong antioxidant and anti-inflammatory Actions which might tone down the damage. Think of Lemongrass and Lemon balm tea not just for the fever but because it is also good for headaches and is Antiviral. In Japan they tested Astragalus for use in Japanese Encephalitis which is another mosquito borne encephalitis, the results were 60 to 80% of infected mice treated survived compared to a 10% survival rate for the untreated. So think of giving Astragalus early in the recovery after the fever is gone.

Hypericum
(St John's Wort)

Actions- Anti-inflammatory, astringent, anti-viral, anti-spasmodic, nervine, vulnerary, antibacterial.

The main reason we are using Hypericum for Murray Valley encephalitis is for it antiviral action and its affinity to the brain along with its pain reducing actions on the nerves.Taken internally has a sedative and pain reducing effect. For neuralgic pain, anxiety, tension, rheumatic pain, sciatica, for pains that shoot along the nerves, as a lotion it will speed the healing of wounds and bruises and is used where there is damage to the nerve rich areas, varicose veins and mild burns. Good for inflamed joints and rheumatic pain. Recently the herb has become popular to use as an antidepressant especially for cases of anxiety. For First Aid use we are concentrating on external use only. Used for wounds with pains that shoot along the nerves, in nerve rich areas such as the fingers, lips, tail bone and toes. As a lotion it will speed the healing of wounds and bruises and is used where there is nerve damage and the possibility of tetanus. The main remedy for puncture wounds. Good for, varicose veins especially the painful kind and mild burns. Patients recovering from surgery where the nerves have been damaged often recover faster with Hypericum. For inflamed joints and rheumatic pain, painful abscesses, bad insect stings, damaged nerves from impact injuries, sprains and ulcers. Eases the pain in conditions such as lumbago, sciatica and Shingles where a cream can be used on the sore and the oil applied along the affected nerve path. As a lotion it is commonly mixed with Calendula, Homoeopaths call this lotion Hypercal. Hypericum has been one of the main Homoeopathic First Aid Remedies for hundreds of years used alone or mixed with Calendula in a solution called HYPERCAL. After the 1930's it faded from popularity, but was used by the Russians in WW2 as a replacement for morphine in Lotion and Potencies

Dose - 1 to 4mls 3 times a day.

Boneset

Eupatorium perfoliatum

Actions - Febrifuge, immune stimulant, diaphoretic, laxative, antispasmodic, anti-inflammatory, and Cholagogue. One of the best remedies for the flu as it relieves the aches and pains as well as dealing with the fever and relieving the mucous congestion of the respiratory tract. Works well in conditions of catarrh such as bronchitis. It can safely be used in any fever and also as a general cleansing agent. Acts on the liver and digestive system increasing bile and helping with constipation. Used for dyspepsia and general debility especially indigestion in the old. Can offer relief in muscular rheumatism and in the past has been used as an anti- malarial. The name Boneset has nothing to do with setting bones but from breakbone fever, as the pain in the bones was so intense it was likened to that of a broken bone, the fever is now known as Dengue fever which is caused by a virus carried by mosquitoes. **Colds and Flu – Think of Boneset for the more severe cases of colds and flus.** This is a good herb to add when the severity of the condition seems to be getting worse especially the fever. Make sure you start to monitor the temperature more frequently especially in the young. **Fever Reducer** - While fever is a natural healing process in the body, over a certain temperature it can become dangerous and even life threatening. Boneset is as a fever reducer which promotes sweat in fevers which act to cool the body down and can remove harmful toxins through the skin. **Immune Boosting** - Boneset has been shown to contain antiviral properties and strengthens the immune system by enhancing the secretion of interferon. Interferons are named for their ability to interfere with viral replication by protecting cells from virus infections. Boneset seems to be effective against minor viral and bacterial infections by stimulating the white blood cells. **Digestive Health** - Boneset can stimulate deficient digestive enzymes in the gastrointestinal tract and also stimulates bile flow from the liver giving a mild laxative effect which allows waste to move through the body more easily. **Cautions** - Should not be used on a long term basis and people with liver problems should be weary. **Parts used** - Whole herb. **Constituents** - Sesquiterpene lactones, polysaccharides, flavonoids, magnesium, calcium, niacin, and phosphorus. **Dose** - Infusion 1 to 2 tsp of dried herb, leave to infuse for 10 minutes and drink as hot as possible (maybe add honey). Tincture – 1 to 2 mls 3 times daily

Homoeopathic Treatment Murray Valley Encephalitis

Aconite 6C to 30C - Nearly all authorities praise this remedy in the early stage especially with a sudden onset where there is high fever, chilliness and dry skin, bounding pulse, thirst, delirium and vertigo to a point. Any noise or light will aggravate the condition.

Belladonna 6c to 30C - Corresponds to the initial stages, where there is intense heat of the body, strong pulse, bright red face and delirium, where the cerebral irritation is marked by intense pain in the head, starting out of sleep crying out, grinding teeth. There are shooting pains in the head which make the patient cringe. These pains are stabbing and come on suddenly and may be accompanied by vomiting. Great irritability.

Hyoscyamus 6C to 30C - Is Suitable for cerebral inflammation with pulsating waves through the head relieved by shaking the head or sitting with the head bent forward. Muscular twitchings, vertigo, brain feels loose, worse at night better stooping.

Stramonium 6C to 30C - This remedy suits inflammatory conditions of the brain with violent delirium. Vertigo is a prominent symptom and also a transient blindness.

Neurasthenia or Chronic Fatigue?

Neurasthenia is the old term used for nervous exhaustion and has been described as, commonly following depressed states or severe illness, which leaves them with a sense of exhaustion and weakness. There is not usually a disease present. Common symptoms for this are fatigue, weakness, headaches, sweating, polyuria, tinnitus, vertigo, inability to concentrate, poor memory, poor sleep, various painful sensations and vaso motor disturbances. This term and condition has been around since the mid-18th century. Following are 2 old formulas and a reasonably new one from Mediherb to who I always pay close attention too. In the past it was also found or thought to be more common in women which is why I think that Wild Yam was chosen in the first and second formula because of the Progesterone content in it, they were probably thinking of hormone balancing. The first birth control pills were made from Wild Yam. Take a good look at the formulas as they are still good for use today. Note that the first 3 have Valerian in them from which the drug Valium comes from. The last more modern formula from Mediherb is using more of the modern herbs called adaptogens which help you adapt and cope better with your condition along with giving you energy so as to function better and start to get on with your life. The adaptogens in this formula are Brahmi, Withania, Ginseng, Siberian Ginseng and Schisandra. I have been working with adaptogens for decades and kind of consider them as friends now, it's nice to use these tools that seem to think of what they need to do, sometimes I even think they are brighter than me. But what else can you expect from an herb named Brahmi, it's obviously a gift from the gods.

Hewlett Parsons Formula - Wild yam, Valerian, Gentian, Skullcap and Mistletoe.

Powells Formula – Skullcap, Valerian, Hops and Wild Yam.

Denis Stewarts Formula - Panax capsules (Ginseng), Oats (nutrition), Hops, Kola, Gentian and Valerian.

Mediherb - Liquorice or Bacopa (Brahmi),Withania, Skullcap, Panax (ginseng), Siberian ginseng, Schisandra and Oil of rosemary.

Chronic Fatigue Syndrome – The Centre for Disease Control and Prevention criteria for chronic fatigue syndrome is a severe fatigue lasting longer than six months, as well as presence of at least four of the following physical symptoms - post exertional malaise, unrefreshing sleep, impaired memory or concentration, muscle pain, polyarthralgia, sore throat, tender lymph nodes, or new headaches. Other symptoms can be a Low grade fever of above 100.4 °F (38°C) and chills, comes on suddenly especially after the flu, Sore throat and swollen lymph glands in the neck or armpits, more common in people over age 40, twice as many women than men are diagnosed with CFS, muscle and joint aches without any swelling, headaches, mood changes, always feels tired, sleep doesn't help, feeling as if you are in a fog and not being able to concentrate or remember and finally the condition can last a month or years. **Cause** – Is still unknown. I think it is very similar to Glandular Fever which I had twice as a teenager and to this day my glands have not gone down. Depression seems to make the condition worse and makes it last longer. I usually think of Astragalus straight away mainly for its anti-viral action. But before starting treatment try to rule out auto immune diseases where the body attacks itself especially if you are thinking of Echinacea which I am, as I want to build up an army of white blood cells to attack and defeat the condition but if it's an autoimmune disease you may just be beating yourself up. With Doctors in this disease you can wind up on anything from anti-depressants to stimulants but one good thing you can do for yourself in this time period is to sort out your diet and get it where it should be. **Nutrition** – Iridology is very useful for trying to sort out this condition and can give you plenty of clues. Some of the main clues I have seen are dark murky clouds in the eyes which suggest a toxic waste dump. These people sometimes have bowel problems and the waste is not getting out so it overloads the other systems such as the liver in trying to get rid of the waste. Some eyes have about 3 or more nerve rings so these people are under constant stress and are rapidly burning calcium and magnesium which is what the nerves live on as well as the B vitamins which are water soluble so they don't stay in the body for long. The last clue from the eye can be what is known as a Lymphatic Rosemary which means the lymph system is not removing waste from the body effectively. Nutrition wise it would be a good idea to use this time to change your diet to what it should be. Avoid refined foods, sugar, caffeine, alcohol, and saturated fats so the body can have a bit of a rest and change to more fresh vegetables, legumes, whole grains, protein, and essential fatty acids found in nuts, seeds, and cold-water fish. See the diet part of the book and go on the acid alkaline diet or even just use the superfoods mentioned there. Omega-3 fatty acids found in fish oil may also help reduce fatigue. Studies show that people with CFS have lower ratios of omega-3 to omega-6 fatty acids. Zinc for the immune system and vitamin C. For a yes or no answer when times get really bad wack the vitamin C up to about 2000 mg and see what happens. Vitamin C is good at getting rid of toxins and rubbish. **Herbal Treatment** – I usually start with Astragalus and Echinacea. Echinacea I would run for 3 months which is the blood cycle and then stop and reconsider the whole case again. For males consider a very low dose like Siberian ginseng which would work more like a tonic. Panax Ginseng basically gives a shot of adrenaline to the blood which could be a bit to brutal. For females consider Withania which is another adaptogen but more female specific but good for anyone, read up about it in the herbal. Lemon Balm can also help in this condition and is also an Antiviral more specific to the nervous system and also used in Glandular Fever, have a read of it in the herbal. Consider Cats Claw if you think there is an Auto immune type of problem floating around in the background. Consider all the formulas old to new given above with the Mediherb Formula being the most modern. As for the answer to the question in the heading I still don't know, but I do know Iridology gives me a better chance to personalize the treatment more and individualize the treatment to certain areas which make me have to think a lot harder instead of treating people as just part of the herd in a 5 minute interview.

Homoeopathic Remedies for Chronic Fatigue Syndrome

Arsenic Album 30C - Patient feels like lying down all the time due to excessive fatigue. Standing, walking and the slightest exertion result in fatigue and lying down provides some relief to the person. Even a little exertion leads to lack of strength and weakness. Such persons also hesitate and have fear exerting because they anticipate exhaustion as a result. Apart from disabling fatigue, anxiety may also show its presence in extreme levels.

Gelsemium 30C - Indicated by weakness with drowsiness, dizziness, dullness and trembling. For mental exhaustion and indifference, physical weakness such as heaviness of the limbs and eyelids. Muscle aches with heaviness and weakness. Tremors and twitching of the muscles may also be a feature. The sufferer might have a dull heaviness in the head and have blurred vision, feels worse in damp, cold weather and mentally be dull with a lot of anxiety. Sleepiness throughout the day with disabling fatigue. Along with drowsiness and fatigue, heaviness in head may also be felt. The muscle pain is mostly present in neck, shoulders, back, hips and legs. The patient may also experience trembling and weakness in limbs.

Kali Phos 30C - A widely used remedy for CFS, especially if the illness follows influenza. The slightest mental or physical exertion leads to extreme fatigue. For such persons, even a little work seems to be a very huge task. Anxiety with depression, insomnia and nightmares. The anxiety may present as a fear of crowds and agoraphobia. Extreme prostration, weakness and tired feeling ensue from a little exertion. The person feels worn out as if all the energy has been drained out. Loss of memory might be a problem. Forgetfulness is noticeable while speaking or writing. There is muscle weakness and aches and pains, all worse with exercise, the cold and mental effort. The symptoms are better from sleep, eating and gentle movement.

Actions Used in the Nervous System

The nervous system touches and joins every part of the body to the brain and when there is something wrong with this system it can have a devastating effect on other parts and produce the worst pains imaginable. One of the most important herbs in this system is

Hypericum also known as St John's Wort. This herb is anti-viral, probably antibacterial, anti-inflammatory, a sedative and one of our main first aid remedies for wounds which helps relieve pain and can kill the tetanus bacteria, this is only mentioning a part of its uses, always consider this herb when there are problems with this system especially if you don't know what the problem is. Another good herb for rebuilding this system is Oats which is a Nervine tonic also think of Valerian which is our main Tranquillizer but also a good tonic for this system. A lot of the herbs mentioned below are used in other systems as well so when you want the action of a Nervine to use in another system try to match the herb to one used in that system as well.

Nervous System Herbs - Brahimi, Chamomile, Cramp bark, Damiana, Gotu Kola, Hypericum, Hops, Hyssop, Linden Flowers, Mistletoe, Passion Flower, Skullcap, Valerian, Vervain

Chamomile

Actions - Antispasmodic, nervine, sedative, carminative, anti-inflammatory, analgesic, antiseptic, allergies.

An excellent gentle sedative with a relaxing action that is good for easing anxiety and helping with sleep. Helps to restore the nervous system. In the digestive system it can be used for indigestion especially when there is colicky pains and is ideal for colitis and IBS type problems. For females Chamomile is good for amenorrhea, spasmodic dysmenorrhea, premenstrual irritability and menopausal tensions. This herb is also a good source of calcium and magnesium which are the nervous systems favorite minerals.

Uses - Anxiety, colic, diverticula's, flatulence, gastritis, indigestion, insomnia, irritable, nervousness, restlessness, stress, ulcers.

Doses - Tincture 2 to 4mls 3 times daily, for teas just the one teabag.

Skullcap

Actions - Nerve tonic, sedative, antispasmodic, stress, anxiety, PMS, anti-depressive, alterative, bitter tonic, cerebral tonic.

Skullcap has a wide range of use mostly focusing on the nerves. It relaxes states of nervous tension while at the same time renewing and revivifying the central nervous system. It has a specific use in the treatment of seizure, epilepsy and hysterical states. It may be used in all exhausted or depressed conditions. Good for easing Pre Menstrual Tension and painful menstruation.

Uses - Alcoholism, arthritis, delirium, convulsions, drug withdrawal, epilepsy, headache, hypertension, nerve pain, panic attacks, Parkinson's disease, restlessness, tremors.

Doses - Tincture 2 to 4mls 3 times a day, 1 to 2 teaspoonful's of dried herb in tea 3 times a day.

Actions for the Nervous System

Antispasmodic - Prevents or eases spasms and cramps.
Herbs - Aniseed, Angelica, Black Cohosh, Chamomile, Fennel, Horehound, Hyssop, Lime Blossom, Mistletoe, Motherwort, Rosemary, Rue, Sage, Skullcap, St John's Wort, Thyme, Valerian, Vervain.

Antidepressive - Damiana, Rosemary, Skullcap, St John's Wort, Valerian, Vervain.

Analgesic - Herbs that reduce pain.
Herbs - Chamomile, Dong Quai, Hops, Ladys Mantle, Passion Flower, St John's Wort, Skullcap, Valerian, Wild Yam, Withania.

Nervine - Has a beneficial effect on the nervous system, acts like a tonic to this system.
Herbs - Black Cohosh, Chamomile, Hops, Lime Blossoms, Mistletoe, Motherwort, Oats, Peppermint, Rosemary, Skullcap, St John's Wort, Tansy, Thyme, Valerian, Vervain, Wormwood.

Sedative - Calms the nervous system and reduces stress and nervousness throughout the body.
Herbs - Black Cohosh, Chamomile, Hops, Hyssop, Motherwort, Skullcap, St John's Wort, Valerian , Vervain.

Diet and Nutrition for the Nervous System and Brain Overview

Here we look at the diets suitable for the nervous system. The main diet I always push is the Acid and Alkaline diet mainly because most of the people I see with cancer or severe chronic diseases when I show them Acid and Alkaline chart they are mainly in the acid side. Next is the MIND Diet that is used for people with or susceptible to brain diseases which is similar to the Mediterranean diet. Following this is the Superfoods for the Nervous System which you should try to use in all the diets.

Diet and Nutrition

As you age you generate less saliva and stomach acid making it more difficult for your body to process certain vitamins and minerals, such as B12, B6 and folic acid, which are necessary to maintain mental alertness, good memory and good circulation. Your taste and smell senses diminishes with age and you lose sensitivity to salty and bitter tastes so you have to be careful not to over salt your food. To all you young ones enjoy it while you can as time tends to go by fast and then it's too late. Time to get back to the basics. First as we age we tend to put on weight because the metabolism is slowing down and food doesn't pass through the system as fast as it used to, which means the body has more time to absorb fat and everything else you don't want it to. For the younger ones you reach your peak at about 36. Next we may not be using as much energy as what we used to for example females after menopause require many hundreds of calories less than before because the body does not need the energy any more to keep the monthly cycle going, so if you are female and in menopause and eat what you have always eaten you will most likely be putting on weight. The benefits of healthy eating include increased mental acuteness, resistance to illness and disease, higher energy levels, faster recuperation times, and better management of chronic health problems, so let's get back to basics. Concentrate buying your food from Vegetable and Fruit shops or the local markets and go back to using the local butcher. Avoid processed foods as they are loaded with the wrong types of fat and too much salt and sugar. Use the supermarket for all your other needs. Just by doing this you are half way there and are keeping a lot of your money in your local community. Malnutrition is your worst enemy as it depletes your body of its reserves and lowers your immune response and the other enemy can be a lower income which is another good reason for going back to basics. Remember the old saying let your foods be your medicines and your medicines be your foods, well now is the time to put it in practice.

Calories needed for adults of different ages.

Use the following as guidelines but remember it is not taking size into account, so big people may need more and little less.

For Women

A woman over 50 who is:

Not physically active needs about 1600 calories a day

Somewhat physically active needs about 1800 calories a day

Very active needs about 2000 calories a day

A woman over 30 to 50 who is:

Not physically active needs about 1800 calories a day

Somewhat physically active needs about 2000 calories a day

Very active needs about 2200 calories a day

A woman over 19 to 30 who is:

Not physically active needs about 2000 calories a day

Somewhat physically active needs about 2000 to 2200 calories a day

Very active needs about 2400 calories a day

For Men

A man over 50 who is:

Not physically active needs about 2000 calories a day

Somewhat physically active needs about 2200 to 2400 calories a day

Very active needs about 2400 to 2800 calories a day

A man over 30 to 50 who is:

Not physically active needs about 2200 calories a day

Somewhat physically active needs about 2400 to 2600 calories a day

Very active needs about 2400 to 2800 calories a day

A man over 19 to 30 who is:

Not physically active needs about 2400 calories a day

Somewhat physically active needs about 2600 to 2800 calories a day

Very active needs about 3000 calories a day

Overview of your new Diet

In reality diets usually don't work. What happens is that people go on a diet then go back to what they normally do and back comes the weight, while our primitive metabolism is thinking wow that was a really bad famine back there, I better store heaps of fat for next year in case there is another famine. The only diets that work are a change in lifestyle and eating habits. As mentioned before get off the processed foods and your half way there. The easiest way to replace old habits is to replace them with new habits, this is the least traumatic way of going about it and at least you will know what the new habits are for. Next is to know yourself and your weaknesses. Regard this statement in the mental and physical. Sticking to the physical and medical point of view we want to make your new diet suited to your weak areas and medical liabilities. You may be genetically programmed and susceptible to cardiovascular disease, Rheumatism and Arthritis or Cancer could be very strong in your family or for male's Prostrate problems, so sticking to your foods being your medicines we want to base your diet on preventing and helping your medical liabilities, but we will go into more detail about that later. Your main focus for your new diet will be low carbohydrate foods, nutritious foods, foods that are high in fibre and moderately lean protein, notice I didn't say lean like all the others do, this is because the high fibre will lower the cholesterol so always remember this for it is one of the main faults of a processed food diet which generally lacks fibre. If you like cooking like me then you know fat is where the flavour is, so where there is animal fat always add fibre and this will lower the cholesterol the body can absorb. Another consideration should be the elimination of refined sugar and refined flour products. Yes I know it's hard but you could do what I do and use honey as my main sweetener its good in teas (sugar substitutes are Stevia, Sorbitol, Allulose, use in small doses)   and as for refined flour, well we all know you can make glue using flour and water, and this is what it does inside of you as well as being responsible for most of the constipation people suffer from. Try to use unrefined preferably organic wholegrain products such as whole meal bread, whole meal flour for cakes, biscuits etc, whole meal pasta, and brown rice.

Protein - Is the building blocks of the body and is required for the ongoing repair of the body. When I used to work in chemists helping people with their dieting I was taught that a general mug proof way of telling people their daily requirements of protein is that it is a palm sized piece of steak or other protein. Minus the fingers and thumb, you want it about the size of the remaining palm and the same thickness of the palm. This is a good and easy way to remember as it suits everyone because a little four foot ladies palm is in proportion to her body, and it's the same for a big seven foot male. It is best to have protein at every meal because protein is hard to digest and requires energy to do so, and when it is all chewed up in the mouth and mixed up with all the other food it forces digestion to go slowly and makes you feel fill longer. Compare this to a simple carbohydrate which is as the name suggests, simple to digest so the body only needs minutes for this and is rewarded with lot of energy. This is the mechanics of the body. Protein rich food being digested has to be digested slower because it is more complex and harder for the body to do, use this to your advantage by having protein with every meal and slow down the digestive process and sugar release, and feel full for longer. This can also save you from Diabetes. The metabolic breakdown of protein produces uric acid so for those with rheumatism, arthritis and gout bear this in mind for a lot of your treatment is aimed at reducing acid so you don't want to go much past your daily requirements. Forms of protein are red meat, poultry, fish, beans, peas, eggs, nuts, seeds, dairy and cheese.

Carbohydrates - Concentrate on the complex carbohydrates rather that the simple carbohydrates, for simple are mainly found in processed foods and release their sugar fast for energy and are part of the reason diabetes is so prevalent now. A good example is white bread. Complex carbohydrates release their sugars slowly because that is what they are complex, so the body has to spend time pulling them to pieces, lots of them are full of fibre which helps to protect us from too much cholesterol and also keeps the bowel moving so complex carbohydrates are a win situation.

Foods to Pay Attention to

Here we will start by explaining what GI is. GI is an abbreviation for Glycaemic Index which is basically the sugar value of each food determined by the rise in blood sugar. High GI is usually found in simple carbohydrates with Low GI found in complex carbohydrates. After the food will be a number which is its GI value, I will start with the high numbers and work down to the low, I am just giving you a small example; you should be able to find lots more low GI foods for your area in the correct seasons.

Low GI = 53 or less

Medium GI = 56 - 69

High GI = 70 or more

Below is just a small list of food to give you ideas, I will leave it to you to research all the low GI foods that you like and match them to your other favourite foods. There are hundreds of books out there that give you the GI of nearly every food there is. Just go through them and choose what you like.

Vegetables - Dark green leafy vegetables are nutrient rich such as spinach and broccoli as well as the yellow and orange vegetables such as carrots, squash and yams. Try to avoid the energy rich ones or high GI ones such as potatoes or eat them in moderation with other complex carbohydrates so as to slow down their sugar release.

Low GI - Sweet corn 47, boiled carrots 41, green peas 39, raw carrots 16, eggplant 15, cauliflower 15, tomatoes 15, green beans 15, broccoli 10, cabbage 10, mushrooms 10, chilies 10, lettuce 10, red peppers 10, onions 10.

Fruits - Try not to have juices as they are generally loaded with extra sugar so focus on whole fruit for the fibre and nutrients especially the more colourful ones as they are usually the ones high in antioxidants.

Low GI - Kiwi fruit 47, coconut 45, grapes 43, pears 41, strawberries 40, oranges 40, apples 34, dried apricots 32, prunes 29, peaches 28, grapefruit 25, plums 24, cherries 22.

Grains - Always go for the whole grains as you get the fibre and they are generally complex carbohydrates so you also get the slow sugar release and stay full longer. White bread has a GI of 71 while soya and linseed bread is 36 GI

Bread Example - Sour dough wheat 54, whole wheat 49, sour dough rye 48, wholegrain pumpernickel 46, heavy mixed grain 45, soya and linseed 36.

Diet, Cancer and Chronic Diseases and Acid

I now believe one of the main causes of cancer is from the body being constantly acidic. It is said Disease and Cancer are found in Acid bodies, it is also said Cancer can't live in an alkaline body. My training as an Iridologist taught me to see what acid eyes look like and the constant contacts of people with cancer over the years slowly lead me to this conclusion. So a long time ago I made my own Acid and Alkaline Chart as it was the only way I could get one at the time. For way over a decade everyone with cancer was shown the chart and we tried to work out where their diet was and nearly all the time they were in the acid areas of the chart or as I refer to it in the acid lane or living in the acid lane. At that time I was in a very large Pharmacy in the middle of a state capital city for a number of years where I had dealings with literally thousands of people with lots of them being tourists. Anyone with cancer was shown the chart and had it explained to them with the result of most of them being in the acid lane, not only in food but usually from stress, worry and overwork. Anger also raises the acid levels and to make it worse I have seen many who are angry at getting Cancer and even more angry that their body has betrayed them, and who's going to look after my young family now. They stand in front of me with their fists clenched tight and you can almost feel the rage, this is not fair, it's not right, what am I going to do, who will look after my family. Using this as an example you can see why you have to remove the cause before any real healing can begin and give them hope. You have to explain to them what their rage and diet is doing to them. Someone with that amount of anger and stress is rapidly using up all their B vitamins, along with calcium and magnesium which the nervous system would be gobbling up at a fast rate, as its taking most of the burden from the stress and then imagine how much adrenaline must be in the blood of one so angry, so that's more B vitamins being used to support that system and a massive raise in blood pressure. Let's move this case further along and see what else is happening. Human blood is always slightly alkaline, if it goes into the acid we die of what is called Acidosis. So if you are living in the acid lane and your blood is in a constant battle to keep itself in the alkaline lane, then the body is in constant stress which makes more acid, but it has no choice but to keep itself-alkaline so to do that it has to use the minerals in the body to buffer that acid, with the main ones being Calcium and Magnesium. Can you see the vicious circle? So imagine a lifetime in the acid lane, living on processed food and fizzy drinks which are pumped full of carbonic acid to make the bubbles and loaded with sugar which breaks down to acid, and you get the sad picture of lots of people with cancer and lots of people with osteoporosis, because the blood has had to steal its Calcium and Magnesium from the bones because it's taken it from every other place as much as it can without breaking down the system. Sometimes the chemist has sent over to me people with cancer who are obviously close to the end of their time and I have shown them the chart, explained it and then given them a photocopy of it and a couple of months later they will pop up and come and see me and say they think it has helped them a bit but by this time it is usually to late the damage is done, but they do appreciate the company and having someone to talk to and I know they will be showing the chart to others and talking about it. Let's now start to get to know the chart. I am happy to say that a lot more people are of the same opinion now so you should be able to find a lot more information on the internet and a few downloadable charts.

Guide to the Chart

Excessively acid bodies try to make themselves more Alkaline so they tend to use what is easily available to do this which is usually Calcium and Magnesium which do a good job of buffering acid. Too much protein puts acid in the system, mainly uric acid which results from the breakdown of protein. White sugar put lots of acid in the body along with alcohol, which when you break it down is just sugar. Disease and Cancer are found in Acid bodies, it is said Cancer can't live in an alkaline body. Use alkaline foods to correct the imbalance. This is what the chart is for, it allows you to see if your diet is to acid and it shows you how to change it by eating more alkaline foods and reducing the acid foods.

1. - Human blood pH should be slightly alkaline (7.35 - 7.45). A pH of 7.0 is neutral. A pH below 7.0 is acidic. A pH above 7.0 is alkaline. A blood pH of 6.9, which is only slightly acidic, can induce coma and death.

2. - An acidic pH can occur from, an acid forming diet, emotional stress, toxic overload, immune reactions or any process that deprives the cells of oxygen and other nutrients. The body will try to compensate for acidic pH by using alkaline minerals. If the diet does

not contain enough minerals to compensate, a build-up of acids in the cells will occur.

3. - Alkaline or Acid forming describes the ash residue after metabolism. Citrus tastes acidic but leaves an alkaline residue.

4. - Disease and Cancer are found in Acid bodies, it is said Cancer can't live in an Alkaline body. Use alkaline foods to correct the imbalance.

5. - Most people eat acid producing processed foods like white flour and sugar and drink acid producing beverages like coffee and soft drinks. We use too many drugs, which are acid forming; and we use artificial sweeteners which really wack up the acid levels.

6. - To maintain health, the diet should consist of 60% alkaline forming foods and 40% acid forming foods. To restore health, the diet should consist of 80% alkaline forming foods and 20% acid forming foods.

7. - Generally, alkaline forming foods include: most fruits, green vegetables, peas, beans, lentils, spices, herbs and seasonings, and seeds and nuts.

8. - Generally, acid forming foods include: meat, fish, poultry, eggs, grains, refined sugar and legumes.

9. - Protein foods combine well with vegetables but not starches. Starches combine well with other vegetables and also light protein such as dairy foods.

10. - Fruit is best on its own. For digestive distress use Lemon juice as this is a great alkalizer.

11. - Try to make the diet 80% alkaline and 20% acid when you start using the chart. Lemon can be added to sauces, casseroles and fish to reduce acid. Nibble on dates etc.

12. - Add lemon juice to the fridge cold water so every time you drink it you are alkalizing the body.

13. - Rest, sleep and exercise are all alkalizers while the negative emotions make acid. Remember to eat according to you occupation.

14. - Deep breathing releases at least 50% of body toxins so set a time aside each day to do this for a while. Remember happy cells don't mutate.

Herbs - Some of the best herbal digestive remedies are Ginger, Peppermint, Chamomile and Dandelion; these can be made as a tea. Apple Cider Vinegar or Lemon can be added to the teas for their alkalizing effect. Foods can be cooked with herbs for those with poor tummies. Think of the mentioned herbs and then add Fennel, Anise, Cayenne, Dill, Garlic, Parsley, Fenugreek, Curry etc. See a Herbalist for Herbs more suited to your condition.

The Acid and Alkaline Chart

For protection against and to help Cancer, Osteoporosis and Chronic Diseases use the Acid and Alkaline Chart. I will repeat this again close to the chart so you can go back and forth easily. Excessively acid bodies try to make themselves more Alkaline so they tend to use what is easily available to do this which is usually Calcium and Magnesium which do a good job of buffering acid. Too much protein puts acid in the system, mainly uric acid which results from the breakdown of protein. Sugar also put lots of acid in the body along with alcohol which also enhances inflammatory conditions. Disease and Cancer are found in Acid bodies, it is said Cancer can't live in an Alkaline body. Use alkaline foods to correct the imbalance. This is what the chart is for, it allows you to see if your diet is to acid and it shows you how to change it by eating more alkaline foods and reducing the acid foods. Diet is very important, consider this, every 3 months the blood replaces itself, every year the bones replace themselves. In a year's time are you going to have a healthy body or a junk food body? Don't forget if you eat on the acid side the bones won't be all that strong anyway.

Extremely Acid Forming Foods - pH 5.0 to 5.5

5.0 - Artificial sweeteners, Overwork, Fear, Stress, Anger, Jealously.

5.5 - Beef, Carbonated soft drinks and fizzy drinks, Cigarettes (tailor made), Drugs, Flour (white, wheat), Goat, Lamb, Pastries and cakes from white flour, Pork, Sugar (white), Beer, Brown sugar, Chicken, Deer, Chocolate, Coffee, Custard with white sugar, Jams, Jellies, Liquor, Pasta (white), Rabbit, Semolina, Table salt refined and iodized, Tea black, Turkey, Wheat bread, White rice, White vinegar (processed).

Moderate Acid - pH 6.0 to 6.5

6.0.-.Cigarette tobacco (roll your own), Fish, Fruit juices with sugar, Maple syrup (processed), Pickles (commercial), Shellfish, Breads (refined) of corn, oats, rice and rye, Cereals (refined) e.g. Weetabix, corn flakes, Wheat germ, Whole Wheat foods, Wine, Yogurt (sweetened).

6.5 - Bananas (green), Buckwheat, Cheeses (sharp), Corn and rice breads, Egg whole (cooked hard), Ketchup, Mayonnaise, Oats, Pasta (whole grain), Pastry (wholegrain and honey), Peanuts, Potatoes (with no skins), Popcorn (with salt and butter), Rice (basmati), Rice (brown), Soy sauce (commercial), Tapioca, Wheat bread (sprouted organic)

Slightly Acid to Neutral pH 7.0

7.0 - Barley malt syrup, Barley, Bran, Cashews, Cereals, (unrefined with honey-fruit-maple syrup), Cornmeal, Cranberries, Fructose, Honey (pasteurized), Lentils, Macadamias, Maple syrup (unprocessed), Milk (homogenized) and most processed dairy products, Nutmeg, Mustard, Pistachios, Popcorn and butter, (plain), Rice or wheat crackers (unrefined), Rye (grain), Rye bread (organic sprouted), Seeds, (pumpkin and sunflower), Walnuts, Blueberries, Brazil nuts, Butter (salted), Cheeses, (mild and crumbly), Crackers (unrefined rye), Dried beans, Dry coconut, Egg whites, Goats milk (homogenized), Olives (pickled), Pecans, Plums, Prunes.

Slightly Alkaline to Neutral pH 7.0

7.0 – Almonds, Artichokes (Jerusalem), Barley-Malt, Brown Rice Syrup, Brussels Sprouts, Cherries, Coconut (fresh), Cucumbers, Eggplant, Honey (raw), Leeks, Miso, Mushrooms, Okra, Olives ripe, Onions, Pickles, (homemade), Radish, Sea salt, Spices, Taro, Tomatoes, (sweet), Vinegar (sweet brown rice), Water Chestnut, Artichoke (globe), Chestnuts (dry roasted), Egg yolks (soft cooked), Goat's milk and whey (raw), Horseradish, Mayonnaise (homemade), Millet, Olive oil, Rhubarb, Sesame seeds (whole), Soy beans (dry), Soy cheese, Soy milk, Sprouted grains, Tofu, Tomatoes (less sweet), Yeast, (nutritional flakes)

Moderate Alkaline - pH 7.5 to 8.0

8.0 - Apples (sweet), Apricots, Alfalfa sprouts, Arrowroot, Flour, Avocados, Bananas (ripe), Berries, Carrots, Celery, Currants, Dates and figs, (fresh), Garlic, Gooseberry, Grapes (less sweet), Grapefruit, Guavas, Herbs (leafy green), Lettuce, (leafy green), Nectarine, Peaches (sweet), Pears, (less sweet), Peas (fresh sweet), Pumpkin (sweet), Sea salt (vegetable), Spinach

7.5- Apples (sour), Bamboo shoots, Beans (fresh green), Beets, Bell Pepper, Broccoli, Cabbage; Cauliflower, Carob, Daikon, Ginger (fresh), Grapes (sour), Kale, Lettuce (pale green), Oranges, Parsnip, Peaches (less sweet), Peas (less sweet), Potatoes and skin, Pumpkin (less sweet), Raspberry, Strawberry, Squash, Sweet corn (fresh), Tamari, Turnip, Vinegar (apple cider)

Extremely Alkaline Forming Foods - pH 8.5 to 9.0

8.5 - Agar, Cantaloupe, Cayenne (Capsicum),Dried dates and figs, Kelp, Limes, Mango, Melons, Papaya, Parsley, Seedless grapes, (sweet), Watercress, Seaweeds, Asparagus, Endive, Kiwifruit, Fruit juices, Grapes (sweet), Passion fruit, Pears (sweet), Pineapple, Raisins, Vegetable juices

9.0 – Lemons and Watermelon.

This was my main chart a long time ago and no doubt there are a few mistakes in it but over time I decided to leave the numbers alone as they can often confuse people and I currently use charts that say HIGHLY ALKALINE, MODERATELY ALKALINE, LOW ALKALINE etc and have lists of foods under each heading. One that I use often now to help people is called Alkaline Food Chart and on another page is Acidic Food Chart and I put them back to back and laminate them which give me an easy to use tool. There are lots to choose from now on the internet; I generally use about 4 of my favourites which give me more foods to choose from. As mentioned before diets don't really work mainly because you soon get back to your old habits when you finish, but this is different as you are doing this for medical reasons and all the foods are natural and healthy and you have the choice to combine them any way you want. As you are not really eating processed foods anymore buy all your fruit and veg locally and use your local butcher and baker and keep all your money in your local community.

The Diet Reality We Live In

The reality is, if you want a healthy diet avoid processed foods. I was reading an article about how the Health System could collapse in the USA because of all the chronic disease in the population and the article ended saying we haven't really got a medical crisis we have a diet crisis. If we fixed the diet there would be no medical crisis. It's amazing how such a simple and obvious truth will probably never be fixed and possibly destroys the Western Worlds Medical system. Let's start with the most obvious problem which is how many people are overweight. The World Health Organization says that 39% of adults aged 18 years and over were overweight in 2016, and 13% were obese. I think we can add at least 3 to 4 percent to that figure at the least to bring it up to modern times. Our western diet of processed foods are loaded with sugar and salt along with nitrates, artificial food colours, preservatives and lots of saturated fats. Salt alone leads to fluid retention which can make it hard to breathe for people with lung problems (only use Vegetable Salt and you will half you dose immediately). We all like fried foods such as chips loaded with fat and salt that can also cause bloating, which pushes the stomach into the diaphragm which crushes the lungs reducing air intake and if you are overweight every time you bend forward your tummy would push into the diaphragm reducing air and possibly causing gastric reflux as well. After Salt and Fat comes the Sugar and we all know what that does, but it is interesting to note that advertising caters to our cravings, which leads to mass production, which then leads to all the processed foods having to be loaded with more chemicals so as to increase their shelf life and make their colours look natural. We are our own worst enemies. One of my biggest gripes about white bread which most of the Western World eats and lives on is that it is nutritionally just carbohydrates for energy. Also consider bread is mostly flour and water (no fibre) which is of course our first glue, and that is exactly what it does inside the body, now known as constipation. When I was a kid I can remember an elderly Maori man telling us, white man is a fool as he grinds the wheat and uses the white flour to make bread and gives all the husks and waste to the Donkeys, now the white men are getting smaller and the donkeys are getting bigger. The reality is if we want to be healthy we first have to get to our right weight. I push the Acid Alkaline diet as it's fairly obvious when you see sick people and investigate their diets they live mostly in the acid lane. This diet gets people back on to natural foods fast and sometimes gives them fast results. Next we will look at some Super Foods that you could add to your own diet.

Drink plenty of Water

This really depends on the climate you are in and what you do for work as a construction worker would need more than an office worker. About 1 and a half to 2 litres a day is a good goal but take lots more on hot days especially in summer. Some people fill a water pitcher every morning with all the water they are supposed to drink in one day and spread it out over the entire day. The human body is made up of 50 to 65 percent of water, which indicates how important it is to the body. Water helps control and regulates our body temperature, keeping it in check so that our brain and vital organs don't overheat or get too cold and maintains the balance of bodily fluids. It allows for the circulation of these fluids within the body, such as our blood, lymph and digestive fluids. Water provides a medium for the body to transport and assimilate nutrients to be used by the body, along with flushing out wastes and toxins via the stool, urine, and sweat. Water is important to our body's ability to function so put your water bottle in the fridge and make sure you slowly get through it during the day. Benefits of keeping your water levels where they should be are a clearer mind and memory, improved digestion, improved energy and less fatigue, a decrease or elimination of headaches, less toxins in the body as water makes them more easier to be flushed out, improved skin complexion, improved bowel regularity and improved cramps or muscle spasms. So always remember water makes everything work better.

Dementia, Alzheimer's, Parkinson's Diet

This write-up refers to the 3 conditions above but here I will refer to them as Dementia because in the end sadly that is what usually happens unless they are lucky enough to die of natural causes. Our main problem here is that most of the damage done to cause these diseases was done a long time ago so we are a bit too late. We are not using this diet to cure dementia, the intent is to slow the disease down and try to reduce or slow down the future deterioration with antioxidants from our Superfoods for the Brain and Nerves and herbs that increase blood supply to the brain such as Ginkgo that will help transport those new antioxidants to the brain along with extra oxygen and nutrients. Our next main tool will be our main day herb which will be **Brahmi** which improves the thinking process during the day and our night herb called **Schisandra** which is my main damaged nerve repair herb which will do the night shift. We want to also get the patient to their right weight, improve fitness and other non-dementia problems. We are expecting that with all this work we should see an improvement in their health and hopefully a slowdown in the onset of the disease. If we can do this and slow the onset of dementia delaying the end stage of dementia as long as we can with the hope that the loved one can die a natural death then having to go through end stage dementia. That I think is about the best we can do but there is always hope for more, maybe in buying time they can find a wonder drug but I doubt it as most drugs are designed to target one thing but in chronic diseases the cause is usually many things. So far we know that Alzheimer's risk factors can be diabetes, obesity and heart disease which our new diet covers fairly well but there are a few other diets out there that we will look at. But always remember it is everything working together that will give us improvements not just one aspect of the treatment alone, what we are doing here is Holistic Medicine with every part doing its work to benefit and improve the whole organism. One of the first diets that they think can help with the dementias is the Mediterranean Diet but I think we all know that one so we will start on the MIND Diet which is a variation of the Mediterranean Diet.

The MIND Diet

This diet came out in 2015 and is based on the Mediterranean diet which emphasizes fruits, vegetables, whole grains, legumes, fish, and other seafood along with unsaturated fats such as olive oils and low amounts of red meat, eggs, and sweets. A variation of this called The MIND Diet focuses on plant-based foods linked to dementia prevention and encourages eating from 10 healthy food groups. This diet limits servings of red meat, sweets, cheese, butter/margarine and fast/fried food. You should easily find this on the internet. Early research suggests that the MIND diet may reduce the risk of Alzheimer's disease and slow the decline in brain function that can happen with age.

Green, leafy vegetables - Aim for six or more servings per week. This includes kale, spinach, cooked greens and salads.

All other vegetables - Try to eat another vegetable in addition to the green leafy vegetables at least once a day. It is best to choose non-starchy vegetables because they have a lot of nutrients with a low number of calories.

Berries - Eat berries at least twice a week - strawberries, blueberries, raspberries and blackberries at least 2 servings a week.

Whole grains - Aim for at least three servings daily. Choose whole grains like oatmeal, quinoa, brown rice, whole-wheat pasta and whole-wheat bread.

Fish - Eat fish at least once a week. It is best to choose fatty fish like salmon, sardines, trout, tuna and mackerel for their high amounts of omega-3 fatty acids.

Poultry - Try to eat chicken or turkey at least twice a week. Fried chicken is not encouraged on the MIND diet.

Beans - Include beans in at least four meals every week. This includes all beans, lentils and soybeans.

Nuts - Try to get five servings of nuts or more each week. Pecans, Flaxseed, Brazil nuts, Almonds, Pumpkin seeds and Walnuts are all good for the heart. Studies have found that higher overall nut intake was linked to better brain function in older age.

Wine - One glass daily. Both red and white wine may benefit the brain.

Olive oil - Use olive oil as your main cooking oil.

Foods to avoid on the MIND Diet

Butter and margarine - Less than 1 tablespoon (about 14 grams) daily. Try using olive oil as your primary cooking fat.

Cheese - Limiting cheese consumption to less than once per week.

Red meat - Three servings each week.

Fried food - The MIND diet highly discourages fried food.

Pastries and sweets - Limit these to no more than four times a week. Researchers encourage limiting your consumption of these foods because they contain saturated fats and trans fats which are found in lots of Processed foods.

The MIND Diet May Reduce Harmful Beta-Amyloid Proteins - may benefit the brain by reducing potentially harmful beta-amyloid proteins which can accumulate and form plaques that build up in the brain, disrupting communication between brain cells and eventually leading to brain cell death.

Summary of the Dementia Diet

1/. Know the energy requirements needed and base the diet around the calories needed.

2/. Consult an Acid and Alkaline chart and try to gauge in which lane the patient has lived their life in. Download 3 or 4 of them for comparison. Adjust diet accordingly.

3/. From all the food lists try to choose ones that they like and will eat.

4/. Have a good look at Superfoods for the Brain and choose what they like. Take a good look at Beans as here you will get Protein and Carbohydrates together.

Possible New Supplement for Dementia

N-acetylecysteine (NAC). It's is looking as though that NAC will prove beneficial for neurodegenerative conditions. The brain neurotransmitter glutamate helps reduce oxidative damage to brain cells associated with aging. Because NAC helps regulate glutamate levels and replenish glutathione, it can help people with brain and memory ailments. Alzheimer's disease slows down a person's learning and memory capacity and research demonstrates NAC may slow the loss of cognitive ability in people with Alzheimer's. Parkinson's disease can also be treated with NAC. As both oxidative damage to cells and a decrease in antioxidant ability contribute to Parkinson's disease, NAC supplements improve both dopamine function and disease symptoms such as tremors. **Warnings** - May slow the rate at which the blood clots and therefore potentially interfere with blood-thinning medications such as warfarin and others. There have been reports of brochospasms caused by NAC in people with asthma so check latest reports and speak with your physician.

Superfoods for the Brain and Nervous System

The brain is an energy intensive organ with a massive work load in running the body and allowing you to think and at the same time walk, work, know your surroundings along with the dangers etc. To do this it uses around 20 percent of the body's calories along with lots of oxygen and a very strong and unimpeded circulation system to carry all its needs in the blood, which is the main transporter. Any problems with energy, oxygen or circulation then you are in trouble. Remember what you eat today walks and talks tomorrow. Here we are looking for the foods good for the heart and brain along with the main actions we need for them which is anti-inflammatory and antioxidants because if the antioxidants can't tone down the bad chemical reactions then the anti-inflammatorys have to deal with the damage fast so as to reduce scar tissue which causes even further damage. After all life's just a chemical reaction that we would rather not think about. We all take our nerves for granted and only think about them when something happens such as you hit your funny bone or start getting cramps, on the whole it's a very reliable system till something goes wrong. A good insurance is to keep them happy with nutrition and their favourites which are Calcium and Magnesium.

Almonds – Nutrient rich and are a good source of monounsaturated fats and fibre that protect against heart disease. Eating almonds will also help you to lower your Cholesterol. Beware that they are also high in calories so only small amounts.

Apples – Apples are low in calories (90) and rich in nutrients and fibre. Eating one medium apple a day may help lower blood pressure, cholesterol, and inflammation. Unpeeled apples are good sources of both fibre and compounds called polyphenols that benefit heart health. The high soluble fibre in apples helps lower cholesterol, while the polyphenols lower blood pressure and stroke risk.

Avocados - Are high in healthy fats, low in sugar and loaded with fibre and potassium. Avocados are a fruit packed with good monounsaturated fats, omega-3, and omega-6 fatty acids that promote healthy blood flow to the brain and support nerves in the brain along with aiding in the absorption of antioxidants. A diet rich with healthy unsaturated fat supports the brain and combats cognitive decline. They contain the digestive enzyme lipase which breaks down fat molecules into smaller fatty acids and glycerol. Although lipase is already made by the body, consuming avocados may ease digestion especially after a high fat meal. Avocados are rich in monounsaturated fats that help keep your heart healthy. Furthermore, the fibre found in avocados is great for digestion and lowering Cholesterol. Avocados help soothe and heal the digestive tract naturally and also contain other enzymes, including polyphenol oxidase which is responsible for turning green avocados brown in the presence of oxygen. The combination of oleic acid, plant sterols, folate and fibre makes for powerful protection from heart disease. One average size of Avocado provides about 975mg of Potassium. Avocados are a good source of folate, vitamin C, vitamin E, vitamin K magnesium, potassium, lutein and copper. The combination of oleic acid, plant sterols, folate, and fibre makes for good protection from heart disease. Think of this as a weekly treat.

Bananas - On top of their digestive enzyme content bananas are a great source of dietary fibre. Bananas can also help to lower your blood pressure as they are high in potassium, magnesium but low in sodium. Bananas are also high in B6 which is a much needed multipurpose vitamin that does not stay in the body long as it is water soluble. So for the cardiovascular system it's the fibre, potassium and magnesium which are going to be of help.

Beans - Beans have been a staple food for thousands of years which many civilizations were built on. Beans are loaded with fibre and protein 25% which makes them nearly a complete food. The most popular dried beans are kidney, black, navy, pinto and lima beans. Red kidney beans are the highest in antioxidants even more then blueberries. Beans are loaded with fibre which reduces cholesterol and folate which is essential for brain function as deficiencies can lead to neurological disorders such as depression and cognitive impairment. Beans contain iron, magnesium, zinc, fibre, antioxidants, and folate.

Beetroot – A good source of folate, rich in potassium, the leafy green tops are rich in beta carotene, calcium and iron. Beetroot and beet greens have been shown to benefit the lungs by optimising oxygen uptake and lung function. Nitrates help relax blood vessels, reduce blood pressure, and optimize oxygen uptake. Beets are also packed with minerals like magnesium and potassium along with vitamin C and carotenoid antioxidants. Beetroot supplements have been shown to improve physical performance and lung function in people with lung conditions, including COPD and pulmonary hypertension, a disease that causes high blood pressure in the lungs. The red pigments in beets contain antioxidants called betalains that has the actions of antioxidant, anti-inflammatory, liver protective and anti-cancer properties.

Berries - New research has shown that in the berries Blackberries have the highest LDL inhibitory effect, followed by red raspberries, sweet cherries, **blueberries** and strawberries, according to Edwin Frankel, Ph.D., of the University of California at Davis where the research was done. **Black Berries** - Are high in beneficial vitamins and minerals, fibre, and antioxidants. They're low in calories, carbs, and fat. One cup of raw blackberries has almost 8 grams of fibre and contains high levels of antioxidants, such as anthocyanins. Antioxidants such as anthocyanins hold many anti-inflammatory and anti-microbial properties. They may also combat diabetes and certain kinds of cancer. New research suggests that an increased intake of blackberries may address obesity by increasing insulin sensitivity and helping the body burn fat more effectively. **Raspberries** are full of fibre and antioxidant polyphenols. **Sweet Cherries** - Just 1 cup of pitted sweet cherries provides 10% of the daily dose for potassium a mineral that is essential for keeping your heart healthy. It's needed to maintain a regular heartbeat and helps remove excess sodium from your body, regulating your blood pressure. They are also rich in powerful polyphenol antioxidants, including anthocyanins, flavonols, and catechins, which may help keep your heart healthy by protecting against cellular damage and reducing inflammation. **Strawberries** are an excellent source of vitamin C. They may also help reduce risk factors for heart disease and control blood sugar.

Blueberries - Are one of the highest berries in antioxidants. The dark blue pigment found in blueberries contains phenols called anthocyanins which are flavonoids with powerful antioxidant capabilities that have been shown to protect tissue from oxidative damage. Blueberries are high in nitric oxide, a molecule that relaxes the inner muscles of blood vessels. This characteristic helps lower blood pressure. They also are a significant source of vitamin C, manganese and are high in soluble fibre which helps your gut remove bile and manage cholesterol; it does this by binding to the cholesterol, salts, minerals, and other bile components and removing it through the body's waste. Good for your eyes to. This fruit may help protect the brain from the damage caused by free radicals and may reduce the effects of age-related conditions such as Alzheimer's or dementia. Antioxidants act against both oxidative stress and inflammatory conditions that can contribute to brain aging and neurodegenerative diseases. Some of the antioxidants in blueberries have been found to accumulate in the brain and help improve communication between brain cells. This effect increases memory, learning, reasoning, decision-making, verbal comprehension, and all cognitive functions. Other rich antioxidant berries are strawberries, black berries, black currants and mulberries. They also supply vitamin C, Manganese and fibre and are known for keeping the brain, heart and blood vessels strong.

Broccoli - Broccoli contains a number of compounds that have powerful antioxidant and anti-inflammatory effects which can help with premature ageing. Broccoli contains compounds that give it anti-inflammatory and antioxidant actions which may help protect the brain. Broccoli is a member of the cruciferous family which also includes cauliflower, brussel sprouts, cabbage, bok choy, and kale. Cruciferous vegetables contain several Glucosinolates which are phytochemicals that reduce your risk of cancer. High glucosinolates can slow the breakdown of the neurotransmitter acetylcholine which we need for the central nervous system to perform properly and keep our brains and memories sharp. Low levels of acetylcholine are associated with Alzheimer's. Broccoli is a superfood because it contains both glucosinolates and large amounts of other nutrients such as calcium, vitamins A, B, C and K, beta-carotene, potassium iron, and fibre. These nutrients protect against free radicals, keep blood flowing well, and remove heavy metals that can damage the brain. Add broccoli to you diet four times each week.

Carrots - Carrots contain vitamin C at about 10 percent of what you need for one day, Vitamin A and many other antioxidants like lycopene. Alongside promoting lung and health, carrots are known to counter the effects of smoking. Loaded with beta carotene it provides protection to smokers who are exposed to an increased risk of numerous cancers and other degenerative diseases. For the heart it is the Potassium and the Fibre where the main benefits come from. Carrots are high in fibre and low in calories, so they're good for weight-loss diets. Vitamin A helps keep your vision healthy. Carrots also supply Biotin which is a B vitamin that plays a role in fat and protein metabolism, Vitamin K1 for blood clotting and vitamin B6.

Coffee - Improves memory and potentially decreases the risk of dementia. Studies suggest that caffeine may also increase the brains capacity for processing information. Caffeine keeps your brain alert by blocking adenosine a chemical messenger that makes you feel sleepy. Coffee is also a source of antioxidants. Studies have linked lifelong coffee consumption with reduced risk of, Cognitive decline, Stroke, Parkinson's disease and Alzheimer's disease.

Dark Chocolate - Dark chocolate is called dark because it contains more cocoa then normal chocolate. Cocoa is rich in natural compounds that are powerful enough to make dark chocolate a superfood. Dose is 1 to 2 ounces of dark chocolate every day but no more, maybe a lot less as it is high in sugar. Cocoa is packed with brain boosting compounds including caffeine and flavonoids which are strong antioxidants that can improve blood flow to the brain and reduce inflammation. Dark Chocolate is rich in magnesium that your body needs for normal nerve and muscle function and provides 5 percent of your daily need of selenium that works as an antioxidant, also contains serotonin, tryptophan, caffeine, theobromine and zinc. A study that included 2,217 participants found that eating chocolate was associated with less atherosclerotic plaque in the coronary arteries. Dark chocolate is rich in polyphenol plant compounds which help increase nitric oxide production and decrease inflammation in the arteries. Studies have also found that eating dark chocolate is associated with a reduced risk of stroke, heart disease, and diabetes.

Dates - Dates are a superfood for the brain and they are also one of our ancient complete foods along with beans as they contain protein. Studies have found dates to be helpful for lowering Iinterleukin 6 in the brain. High levels are associated with risks of neurodegenerative diseases like Alzheimer's. In animal studies it has been shown dates can be helpful in reducing the activity of amyloid beta proteins which can form plaques in the brain and reduce nerve transmissions which may lead on to Alzheimer's disease. Dates are loaded with antioxidants, vitamins and minerals. A 100 gram serving of dates give you 75g of carbs, 7g of fibre, 2g of protein, 20 percent of the RDI of potassium, 14 percent of the RDI of magnesium, 18 percent of the RDI of copper, 14 percent of the RDI of manganese, 5 percent of the RDI of iron, 12 percent of the RDI of B6 which is one of our main brain vitamins. Dates are high in antioxidants with the main ones being Flavonoids, Carotenoids and Phenolic acid known for its anti-inflammatory properties.

Eggs - Choline is an important micronutrient that your body uses to create acetylcholine, a neurotransmitter that helps regulate mood and memory and is also used for conditions such as Alzheimer's disease, Huntington's disease, mania, memory problems and depression. One egg gives you a quarter of the daily dose. It also helps with blood pressure and hardening of the arteries. It is found in the egg white and also in beans, liver, milk, peanuts and yeast. Eggs are also a good supply of B6, B12 and folate which all do important work in the brain.

Green Tea - Here like coffee it's the caffeine's effect on the brain. Another is L-theanine which is an amino acid that can cross the blood-brain barrier and increase the activity of the neurotransmitter GABA, which helps reduce anxiety and makes you feel more relaxed by strangely countering caffeine. Green tea is also rich in polyphenols and antioxidants that could protect the brain from mental decline and reduce the risk of Alzheimer's and Parkinson's disease.

Mixed Nuts and Seeds – Nuts and seeds are good for the brain as these foods contain omega-3 fatty acids and antioxidants along with being loaded with nutrients. Remember nuts are seeds so they have to be loaded with nutrients so as to give the plant the best start it can which is also why they are usually loaded with calories. Nutrients in nuts such as healthy fats, antioxidants and vitamin E have beneficial effects on brain health. Walnuts may have an extra edge since they contain anti-inflammatory omega-3 fatty acids. When you take the walnut out of the shell what does it look like? Maybe it's trying to tell you something. Pecans, Flaxseed, Brazil nuts, Almonds, Pumpkin seeds and Walnuts are all good for the heart. Studies have found that higher overall nut intake was linked to better brain function in old age. Nuts and seeds are rich sources of the antioxidant vitamin E, which protects cells from oxidative stress caused by free radicals. Research has found that vitamin E may also contribute to improved cognition and reduced risk of Alzheimer's disease.

Oats and Oatmeal – This wholegrain is full of soluble fibre which prevents the body from absorbing cholesterol. Beta-glucan fibre in oats is effective at reducing both total and LDL cholesterol levels and may increase the release of cholesterol rich bile from the liver. The antioxidants in oats also have anti-inflammatory properties which can help reducing inflammation in the arteries. Rolled oats are good but steel cut oats are better as they have more fibre and the fibre is denser.

Oranges - Oranges are loaded with vitamin C which is one of the main antioxidants. One orange contains about 80mg of Vitamin C so an orange a day would cover your daily needed dose. Oranges contain calcium, folate and are high in potassium which is a mineral that regulates heartbeat and muscle function and has also been shown to lower blood pressure. Hesperidin is a citrus flavonoid that's one of the main antioxidants in oranges and may have blood pressure-lowering, anti-inflammatory, and antioxidant effects in the body. Hesperidin is also used for blood vessel injuries especially in large bruises.

Extra Virgin Olive Oil – Consuming more than half a table spoon of olive oil a day may lower the heart disease risk a 2020 study found. Olive oil is one of the key components of the Mediterranean diet which is well known for its heart health. Olive oil is rich in monounsaturated fat which helps lower the harmful LDL cholesterol. When olive oil replaces saturated fat like butter it can help lower cholesterol levels. As the oil was cold pressed without heat and chemicals all the polyphenols where saved.

Pumpkin Seeds - Contain powerful antioxidants that protect the body. These seeds are loaded with zinc, iron, copper, magnesium, manganese, phosphorus and vitamin K. They also contain a lot of antioxidants and a decent amount of polyunsaturated fatty acids and vitamin B2. Pumpkin seeds are full of antioxidants that may help protect against disease and reduce inflammation. They are also used to treat high blood pressure and high blood sugar. It is the high magnesium and potassium that make it good for the heart and blood pressure and nerves. Because pumpkin seeds are high in calories only have about one quarter cup a day.

Spinach - Spinach is a leafy green vegetable rich in nutrients but low in calories and can be eaten raw or cooked. Spinach can be bitter but is less so when cooked. Spinach is high in potassium which helps the electrical conductivity of the brain and also helps the heart by keeping your heart beating at the right pace and keeping the blood pressure down. It does this by helping to control the electrical signals of the myocardium. The folate in spinach reduces homocysteine levels that are associated with an elevated risk of cardiovascular disease. Contains vitamin C, vitamin K, and vitamin A in the form of carotenoids, vitamin B1, vitamin B2, vitamin B6, vitamin E, manganese, folate, magnesium, copper, calcium, potassium, dietary fibre, phosphorus, zinc, protein and choline.

Soy Products – Eating tofu and other soy based products can lower your risk of cardiovascular diseases, coronary heart disease and Strokes along with some cancers. Eating Soy protein such as tofu, tempeh and miso rather than animal meat helps lower the cholesterol levels. One study found that as little as 20g of soy protein per day is effective in reducing total cholesterol while another study found that soy can help reduce triglyceride levels. Soy has been a staple in the diet for many Asian countries such as Japan and has proved its health benefits. It's a complete protein and is rich in fibre and omega-3 fatty acids, plus contains essential vitamins and minerals and many antioxidants.

Salmon and Fatty Fish - What makes oily fish so good is that they contain active fats in a ready-made form which means the body can use it easily. Essential fatty acids (EFAs) cannot be made by the body so they must be obtained through our diet. The most effective one omega-3 fats occur naturally in oily fish in the form of EPA and DHA. A diet with higher levels of these fats may help in lowering the risks of dementia, Alzheimer's disease, and also slow mental decline as well as helping heart and circulation health. Salmon, trout, tuna, herring and sardines are all good rich sources. About 60% of your brain is made of fat, and half of that fat is comprised of omega-3 fatty acids. Your brain uses omega 3 to build brain and nerve cells and these fats are essential for learning and the memory. For brain health two servings of fish per week are recommended. Fish oil is good for other inflammatory diseases such as Rheumatism and Arthritis. Fish with the highest amount of these good oils always live in the coldest waters. If you don't like fish you could invest in some Fish Oil Capsules the EPA and DHA content should be written on the label.

Tomatoes - Tomatoes and tomato products are among the richest dietary sources of lycopene. Lycopene is a powerful antioxidant with many health benefits such as a cancer-fighter lowering the risk of certain types of cancers particularly for bone, lung, and prostate cancers. Is of benefit to heart health as a recent study found evidence that lycopene reduced bad cholesterol (LDL) while increasing good cholesterol (HDL) levels. Lycopene may be most effective when consumed from rich foods like tomatoes and other red or pink fruits. And because they're low in calories and low in sugar they are ideal to add to a heart healthy diet.

Whole Grains - The body needs energy and gets it from glucose in our blood. It's best to supply this by choosing whole grains which give a slow sugar release into the bloodstream. White bread, white sugar and other refined sugars give a far too big rush of sugar which overwhelms the body, eventually leading to diabetes. Too much sugar flowing through the arteries along with the wrong types and unnatural fats, damages the whole circulatory system especially the arteries and prematurely ages the whole system. The slow release of sugars by whole meal and grain products keeps our brains alert throughout the day. Whole grains also provide vitamin E which helps with heart health. Whole-grain foods are brown rice, barley, bulgur wheat, oatmeal, whole-grain bread and pasta. Carbs are often considered the enemy when it comes to health, but whole grains are rich in complex carbohydrates, fibre, and some omega-3 fatty acids that shield the heart from damaging sugar spikes, cholesterol, blood clots, and more. Grains also contain B vitamins that have an effect on blood flow to the brain and mood. Whole grains should be soaked, fermented, sprouted, or grown as sprouts to unlock all their nutritional power.

Nutrition for the Nerves

The 5 Star Super Foods are - Grapes, Millet, Wheat germ, Brewer's Yeast, Oats, Buckwheat and Molasses

Other Super Foods

Fruit - Apricots, bananas, dates, oranges, apples, pears, plums, grapes, peaches, blackcurrants, lemons, figs, strawberries, raspberries.

Vegetables - Asparagus, avocado, aubergine, beetroot, cabbage, carrots, celery, chicory, watercress, French beans, lettuce ,turnip, onions, leeks.

Grains - Oats, barley, rye, whole wheat, wheat germ, brown rice, buckwheat.

Seeds and Nuts - Almonds, pecans, walnuts, sunflower seeds, pumpkin seeds, sprouted seeds.

Legumes - All dried beans, Soya beans, dried peas, sprouted beans,

Herbs and Spices - Garlic, parsley, lemon balm, basil, rosemary, camomile, ginger root, thyme, nutmeg, juniper berries, liquorice, marjoram.

Others - Cockles, shrimps, oysters, sardines, liver, kidney, lean beef, egg yolks.

The Danger Foods

Refined Carbohydrates - White flour and white sugar and processed foods should be avoided.

Alcohol - Only in moderation as large amounts breaks down the B complex vitamins and also has a devastating impact on the stores of magnesium, zinc and calcium.

Aluminium- Avoid using aluminium pans, kettles, teapots and coffee percolators as this metal is highly toxic and accumulates in the body and has been linked to Alzheimer's disease.

Tonic Herbs for This System - Chamomile, Hops, Oats, Valerian, Gotu Kola.

Nervous System Herbal

Astragalus
Astragalus membranaceus

Actions - Immuno-modulator, anti-viral, adaptogen, hypotensive, immune stimulant, adrenal tonic, diuretic, vasodilator, cardiotonic, antioxidant, hepatoprotective, hypoglycemic.

This herb is usually used in chronic diseases as a preventative or in cases of fatigue especially in chronic diseases. Stimulates the natural production of interferon and intensifies the white cell destruction of germs. A good tonic for strengthening the resistance to disease. Is very useful for chronic debility and fatigue by restoring the immune function. Use as a lung tonic to help expel toxins and pus in flu's, colds and sinusitis. Increases stamina and can accelerate wound healing, can help to replenish bone marrow. Strengthens the digestive system and aids adrenal gland function. This herb is used for cancer especially if the patient has had chemotherapy and helps aid them in their recovery. Thought to control body fluids such as excessive sweating, night sweats and relieve fluid retention. Astragalus has powerful anti-aging properties slowing the aging process at a cellular level. Astragaloside IV a saponin has shown benefits in reversing cell damage and in activating telomerase, this addresses telomere shortening and slows down cellular aging. This is very important, I will try to explain. Inside every cell of your body is a Telomere, a good way to think about it is as an hour glass. Every time a cell divides it breaks a little piece of the telomere off which is a bit of sand flowing through the hour glass, when the last piece of the telomere is gone that is the last time the cell can divide, this is how we age. Now I will explain why Antioxidants are so important. Imagine a nasty little free radical with a baseball bat which has just smashed into one of your cells and is wandering round inside and then comes across the telomere and says I will fix you and smashes the telomere right at the bottom and leaves only a little stump left. That's it for the cell, life has been cut short. Astragalus root is most effective when taken long term, providing many benefits that can contribute to a longer, healthier life. Good to use for chronic fatigue syndrome (CFS) and fibromyalgia. Has cardio protective affects helping to prevent plaque buildups in the arteries and narrowing of the blood vessel walls, by protecting the inner wall of the vessel. It has also been shown to reduce blood pressure and lower triglycerides. **Immune Boosting -** Is an immune stimulant that it is known to increase the count of white blood cells and stimulate the production of antibodies, this builds up bodily resistance to viruses and bacteria. Many clinical studies have shown it boosts the immune system and encourages an increase in immune T-cells, natural killer cells, macrophages and immunoglobulin activity, production, and function. Astragalus appears to trigger immune cells from a resting state into heightened activity. The natural killer cells of the immune system also seem to be markedly enhanced to fight intruders five to six times higher than normal. **Cautions** - Should not be used in acute infections or fevers. Use with care for those with very low blood pressure. Women who are pregnant or breastfeeding should not use Astragalus. May counteract anti-diabetic agents, and potentiate effects of diuretics. People with autoimmune diseases should consult their healthcare professional before using Astragalus because of its ability to stimulate the immune system. **Part used -** Root **Dose** - 500 to a 1000mg per day or up to 20 drops of tincture twice daily.

Black Cohosh
Cimicifuga racemosa

Actions - Emmenagogue, anti-spasmodic, nervine, alterative, sedative, tonic, anodyne, vasodilator.

Black Cohosh has a normalizing action on the balance of female sex hormones and may be safely used to regain normal hormonal activity that should give relief to Menopause symptoms. This would be the herb for you if you also suffered from rheumatism or arthritis. Has hormone balancing properties, ovarian cramps or cramping pain in the womb, used to regain normal hormone activity, good for hot flashes, muscular and neuralgic pains with a good example being Sciatica. Black Cohosh may also lower blood pressure, lower cholesterol, help with insomnia and help with tinnitus. Regarded as a relaxing nervine. **Doses-** For tincture is 2-4mls 3 times a day, One and a half teaspoonful's for tea 3 times a day. **Cautions**- Best taken with meals so as to avoid any chance of upsetting tummy. Allow up to 8 weeks to see benefits in menopausal problems and even then the full benefit of the herb may not be reached till 6 months' time. Antibiotics can reduce the effect of this herb.

Brahmi
Bacopa

Actions - Adaptogen, aterative, anti-inflammatory, antioxidant, cognition and memory enhancer, nerve tonic, mild sedative and anticonvulsant, anti-aging.

Used for increasing brain function, or promoting longevity, cerebral circulatory tonic. Central nervous system restorative. Relaxant to the whole nervous system. Has a reputation for enhancing circulation to the brain, thereby increasing short and long-term memory, improving concentration, mental performance & cognitive function as a whole. Used in disorders of the nervous system such as insomnia, anxiety, stress, stroke, Alzheimer's and Parkinson's disease.

Boneset
Eupatorium perfoliatum

Actions - Febrifuge, immune stimulant, diaphoretic, laxative, antispasmodic, anti-inflammatory, and Cholagogue. One of the best remedies for the flu as it relieves the aches and pains as well as dealing with the fever and relieving the mucous congestion of the respiratory tract. Works well in conditions of catarrh such as bronchitis. It can safely be used in any fever and also as a general cleansing agent. Acts on the liver and digestive system increasing bile and helping with constipation. Used for dyspepsia and general debility especially indigestion in the old. Can offer relief in muscular rheumatism and in the past has been used as an anti- malarial. The name Boneset has nothing to do with setting bones but from breakbone fever, as the pain in the bones was so intense it was likened to that of a broken bone, the fever is now known as Dengue fever which is caused by a virus carried by mosquitoes. **Colds and Flu – Think of Boneset for the more severe cases of colds and flus.**

This is a good herb to add when the severity of the condition seems to be getting worse especially the fever. Make sure you start to monitor the temperature more frequently especially in the young. **Fever Reducer** - While fever is a natural healing process in the body, over a certain temperature it can become dangerous and even life threatening. Boneset is as a fever reducer which promotes sweat in fevers which act to cool the body down and can remove harmful toxins through the skin. **Immune Boosting** - Boneset has been shown to contain antiviral properties and strengthens the immune system by enhancing the secretion of interferon. Interferons are named for their ability to interfere with viral replication by protecting cells from virus infections. Boneset seems to be effective against minor viral and bacterial infections by stimulating the white blood cells. **Digestive Health** - Boneset can stimulate deficient digestive enzymes in the gastrointestinal tract and also stimulates bile flow from the liver giving a mild laxative effect which allows waste to move through the body more easily. **Cautions** - Should not be used on a long term basis and people with liver problems should be weary. **Parts used** - Whole herb. **Constituents** - Sesquiterpene lactones, polysaccharides, flavonoids, magnesium, calcium, niacin, and phosphorus. **Dose -** Infusion 1 to 2 tsp of dried herb, leave to infuse for 10 minutes and drink as hot as possible (maybe add honey). Tincture – 1 to 2 mls 3 times daily

Cat Mint
Nepeta cataria

Actions - Carminative, antispasmodic, diaphoretic, sedative, astringent.

This herb is also known as Catnip. Cats and other creatures eat this plant and also give themselves a massage in it. This is an old traditional cold and flu remedy especially for ones with fever. Has an action on the digestive system easing stomach upsets, dyspepsia, wind and colic. Used for diarrhea of the young. Good for the nervous, stressed or restless, helps stomachaches by calming the nerves, used for stress and nervousness. **Dose** - 2 to 4mls of tincture 3 times a day. Good for teas.

Chamomile
Matricaria recutita

Actions - Antispasmodic, nervine, sedative, carminative, anti-inflammatory, analgesic, antiseptic, allergies.

An excellent gentle sedative with a relaxing action that is good for easing anxiety and helping with sleep. Helps to restore the nervous system. It is safe to use in children and is a powerful anti-inflammatory in almost any condition and a good all round tonic for the nervous system. This is the herb for those that can worry themselves sick. As a relaxant, chamomile depresses the central nervous system, reducing anxiety while not disrupting normal performance or function. Chamomile has been used for centuries to lower pain and reduce inflammation. This seems to be backed up by science with a 2009 study finding that chamomile caused cell reactions similar to that of nonsteroidal anti-inflammatory drugs. In the digestive system it can be used for indigestion especially when there is colicky pains and is ideal for colitis and IBS type problems. For females Chamomile is good for amenorrhea, spasmodic dysmenorrhea, premenstrual irritability and menopausal tensions. This herb is also a good source of calcium and magnesium which are the nervous systems favorite minerals. **Uses** - Anxiety, colic, diverticula's, flatulence, gastritis, indigestion, insomnia, irritable, nervousness, restlessness, stress, ulcers. **Doses -** Tincture 2 to 4mls 3 times daily, for teas just the one teabag.

Cowhage
Macuna Pruriens

Actions – Adaptogen, Nerve Tonic, Diuretic, Aphrodisiac, Alterative and Hypotensive.

Mucuna Pruriens is beneficial to brain health as its primary compound levadopa (L-dopa) is a precursor to dopamine, adrenaline and noradrenaline. L-dopa is synthesized in the brain into dopamine which is often used as a treatment in Parkinson's disease. While dopamine is commonly associated with pleasure it actually plays a critical role in muscle control. By raising low dopamine levels this herb can have a positive effect on motivation, attention span and the ability to relax and general mental well-being. As an Adaptogen the herb contains a unique set of phytonutrients that feed the adrenals, balance hormones and significantly reduce stress levels by lowering cortisol. Its libido enhancing effects are thought to be due to the high levels of L-dopa which converts into dopamine in the body. In Brazil the seed has been used internally for Parkinson's disease and other forms of tremors, oedema, impotence, intestinal gas, and worms. It is also considered a diuretic and nerve tonic. Used in Central America as a coffee substitute, whilst in certain parts of Guatemala it is a staple food in tribal diets. Chinese Medicine uses it as an enhancing herb and a prized herb for longevity as well as being a powerful aphrodisiac and adaptogenic herb. **Precautions** - Cowhage can interact with other medications such as those taken for diabetes, antidepressants and antipsychotics. It can also lower blood pressure. **Dosage** - Tincture 2 to 5ml up 3 times daily. Powder form 1 teaspoon up to 3 times daily

Damiana
Turnera diffusa

Actions - Nerve tonic, antidepressant, laxative, urinary antiseptic, stomachic.

Strengthening remedy for the nervous system, tonic action on hormone system, for anxiety and depression especially with a sexual association, tonic to the male reproductive system for impotence, anxiety and neurosis. Tonic for the aged especially in senile decay. For males it is specially indicated for alleviating problems of achieving and maintaining erections. Damiana also works to relieve stress and anxiety related to fears of inadequate sexual performance. One of the active constituents of this herb is thymol which is a compound that is responsible for Damiana's life enhancing and stimulating effect on the mind and body. Used for mild to moderate depression, anxiety and nervous exhaustion. Its stimulating and restorative properties make it a valuable herb for anxiety and depression occurring together as can often happen as a result of long term stress. **Contraindications** – Pregnancy. **Parts Used** – Leaves, **Pharmacy:** Infusion: 1 tsp/cup water, TID. Tincture: (1:5, 60%), 1-2 ml

TID. **Toxicity** - None reported. **Dose** – Tincture 1 to 2 mls 3 times daily. Infusion 1 teaspoon full to cup of boiling water.

Echinacea
Echinacea angustifolia

Actions - Immune stimulant, anti-microbial, anti-inflammatory, alterative, healing.

This herb is an infection fighter active against strep bacteria (abscesses and boils), a blood cleanser, (blood poisons, snake bites, poisonous insects) and a glandular and lymphatic system cleanser. Use it particularly for respiratory infections and for any disease above the waist. This is one of our main immune boosters for the acute diseases. Echinacea stimulates the bone marrow to make more white blood cells which are our main infection killers and why we only use it in short bursts. Use as a prophylactic to protect from infections especially when traveling or before going into Hospital. **Uses** - All infections, depressed immune function, inflammatory conditions, allergies, effective against both bacteria and viruses. **Dose** – 1 to 4mls of tincture. **Warning** - Do not use continually as you will burn out the immune system give a few weeks break after 3 weeks. Beware also in the use of allergies for you could be building up the immune system just to attack itself.

Feverfew
Tanacetum parthenium

Actions - Analgesic, anti-inflammatory, emmenagogue, vasodilator, relaxant, digestive bitter, febrifuge, uterine stimulant.

Alleviates pain, headaches and inflammation and is similar to aspirin but stronger with a slower effect. Research has shown that feverfew inhibits the release of histamine from mast cells and inhibits the production of leukotrienes. Decreases inflammation in blood vessels and in arthritic conditions as well as increases menstrual flow and induces menstruation. The bitters stimulate appetite and improve digestion and kidney function. One of the main remedies used for migraines, especially those that are relieved by applying warmth to the head. Feverfew contains a chemical called parthenolide which helps relieve smooth muscle spasms and can combat the widening of blood vessels that occurs in migraines. Feverfew can reduce the frequency of migraines and reduce symptoms such as nausea, vomiting and sensitivity to light. The bitters in Feverfew stimulate appetite and improve digestion. It is one of the most important aids for female ailments especially in menstrual cramps which occur when the lining of the uterus makes large amounts of prostaglandins when breaking these cells down during menstruation, the prostaglandins are released constricting the blood vessels in the uterus causing painful cramps. Increases menstrual flow and induces menstruation. Feverfews anti-inflammatory actions help to prevent swelling and damage to the joints in arthritis. **Contraindications** - Pregnancy due to emmenagogue effects. **Interactions** - May interfere with anti-coagulant medications. **Dose** - 3 to 4mls of tincture 3 times daily. For tablets take dosage on pack.

Garlic
Allium sativum

Actions - Immune stimulant, anti-bacterial, anti-viral, anti-fungal, anti-septic, anti-oxidant, diaphoretic, cholagogue, hypotensive, anti-spasmodic, vermifuge and many more.

The plant is rich in volatile oil and Sulphur and because of its remarkable penetrating, disinfecting and mucous expelling powers garlic is a valuable basic remedy for the treatment of all ailments in which the cleansing of the blood stream and expulsion of mucous accumulations is required. Garlic is one of our main herbs used to prevent and treat respiratory infections. Anyone who has had garlic breath has experienced this herb's aromatic compounds being excreted through their lungs which is why garlic's active ingredients can be so effective for respiratory complaints. Garlic is extremely effective in dissolving and cleansing cholesterol from the blood stream, it stimulates the digestive tract, kills worms, parasites and harmful bacteria, normalizes blood pressure and reduces fever, gas and cramps. I use Garlic in oil form (Garlic Oil Capsules) for respiratory infections as the oil goes into the blood stream fast and a lot of it exits via the lungs hence the garlic breath. **Uses -** All infections, coughs, colds, flu, bronchitis, all fevers, pulmonary conditions, gastric and skin complaints, rheumatism, all worms and ringworm, ticks and lice. Acts on Bacteria, Viruses and Internal Parasites. **Dose –** 3000mg Garlic Oil tabs are the best way to go as it gets into the blood fast. For those who cannot tolerate the breath use Kyloc the Japanese aged form as this is odorless.

Ginger

Actions - Carminative, anti-inflammatory, vasodilator, stimulant, diaphoretic, anti-emetic.

The therapeutic benefits of ginger are largely due to its volatile oil and oleoresin content. Its antiseptic properties also make it beneficial for gastro-intestinal infections. Aids in fighting colds, colitis, digestive disorders, wind, increases saliva, is excellent for the circulatory system and helps increase stamina and it is also commonly used to help the other herbs in a formula to get into the body. On top of this ginger has a strong antioxidant action that may also help to tone down the inflammatory response. Other uses are for indigestion, nausea, feverish conditions especially when chills are present, travel sickness especially sea sickness, dyspepsia, colic and flatulence.

Dose - Weak tincture 1.5 to 3mls 3 times daily, Ginger tea, crystallized ginger.

Ginkgo Biloba
Maidenhair tree

Actions - Anti fungal, anti-bacterial, antioxidant, cerebral tonic, circulatory stimulant, anti-allergy and anti-inflammatory but mainly used for its Peripheral Vaso - Dilator effects.

Is native to Northern China and is considered the world's oldest tree species. Due to its effect on peripheral and cerebral (brain) circulation it can assist the blood supply to limbs (cramping) and head with the extra oxygen and glucose increasing general alertness. The leading symptoms pointing to Ginkgo are cold hands and feet. This herb opens up the femoral arteries and neck arteries increasing blood supply to those areas thus improving the function of everything in those areas by the increase in oxygen, blood sugar and nutrients. For some, thinking and seeing may improve and walking can also become a bit easier. In asthma Ginkgo helps reduce the inflammation response making the attacks less severe. The herb is safe to use as a tonic. This is a good herb to take in a mixed antioxidant formula. Its strong antioxidant effects are useful in peripheral vascular disease and restricted blood flow for any reason. Good for age related physical and mental deterioration, including Alzheimer's disease and senile dementia and cardiovascular disease along with cerebral vascular insufficiency and impaired cerebral performance. The ability of gingko to strengthen blood vessels, combined with decreased blood clotting leads to better circulation and reduced inflammation, both of which are beneficial to a healthy heart. **Contraindications -** Use caution with patients on anticoagulant or anti-platelet medication such as warfarin and aspirin, in cases of excessive bleeding, or within 14 days prior to surgery. **Dose-** This is easy to find now so dose as on the container. It is now often now combined with Brahmi so as to improve thinking. Tincture – 2 to 4 mls 3 times daily.

Hawthorn
Crataegus oxycantha

Actions - Cardiac tonic, hypotensive, adaptogen, anti-oxidant, coronary vasodilator.

Strengthens the muscles and nerves of the heart, aids in relieving emotional stress, regulates high and low blood pressure, and helps combat arteriosclerosis and heart disease. Strengthens the contractive force of the heart and gently dilates and relaxes the coronary blood vessels. Increases the body's ability to utilize oxygen. This is more of a balancing herb hence the name adaptogen, if the blood pressure is high or low the herb will balance it, if the electrical activity is playing up with rapid or erratic heart beat it will try to balance it which is why it is called an adaptogen. Strengthens and helps to remove plaques from the blood vessels. This is an herb for taking long term. As a long-term treatment may be used safely in heart failure (cardiac insufficiency) and weakness. May similarly be used in cases of palpitations, arrhythmia and valvular insufficiency. Will play a role in any treatment of vessel problems including varicose veins or even ulcers. For blood pressure alone add about 500mg daily of magnesium as this can improve the treatment especially if part of the problem is stress. **Heart Failure** - Hawthorn Berries have been extensively studied in relation to congestive heart failure, with findings concurring that symptoms such as shortness of breath and tiredness can be dramatically improved. One study found that 900mg daily of Hawthorn Berry extract was as effective at managing the symptoms of congestive heart failure as its pharmaceutical counterpart. The flavones enhance the function of cardiac enzymes which can improve the heart's ability to withstand stress. **Angina -** Sufferers can greatly benefit from this herb. One study found that 100mg of Hawthorn extract taken 3 times a day decreased angina in 91% of the participants. It is thought this effect is down to the ability of Hawthorn to increase blood flow to the heart by dilating both peripheral and coronary blood vessels. **Toxicity -** No adverse effects expected within recommended doses. **Interactions -** May help reduce toxicity of cardiac glycosides, hypertensive medications and CNS depressants. **Uses-** As a tonic to the circulatory system and to strengthen the heart for at least 2 months. **Dose** - 2 to 4mls of tincture 3 times a day. Hawthorn Berries - 1 to 2 tea spoons full in cup boiling water up to 3 times a day.

Hypericum
(St John's Wort)

Actions- Anti-inflammatory, astringent, anti-viral, anti-spasmodic, nervine, vulnerary, antibacterial.

Taken internally has a sedative and pain reducing effect. For neuralgic pain, anxiety, tension, rheumatic pain, sciatica, for pains that shoot along the nerves, as a lotion it will speed the healing of wounds and bruises and is used where there is damage to the nerve rich areas, varicose veins and mild burns. Good for inflamed joints and rheumatic pain. Recently the herb has become popular to use as an antidepressant especially for cases of anxiety. For First Aid use we are concentrating on external use only. Used for wounds with pains that shoot along the nerves, in nerve rich areas such as the fingers, lips, tail bone and toes. As a lotion it will speed the healing of wounds and bruises and is used where there is nerve damage and the possibility of tetanus. The main remedy for puncture wounds. Good for, varicose veins especially the painful kind and mild burns. Patients recovering from surgery where the nerves have been damaged often recover faster with Hypericum. For inflamed joints and rheumatic pain, painful abscesses, bad insect stings, damaged nerves from impact injuries, sprains and ulcers. Eases the pain in conditions such as lumbago, sciatica and Shingles where a cream can be used on the sore and the oil applied along the affected nerve path. As a lotion it is commonly mixed with Calendula, Homoeopaths call this lotion Hypercal. **How To Use -** Use as a Lotion one part tincture to twenty parts water to wash out wounds or medicate affected area, make at 1 to 10 for painful and dirty wounds. Mix with Calendula in large painful bleeding wounds with a chance of tetanus. Use Tincture for medicating creams. **History -** St. John's Wort has enjoyed a reputation as a wound healer since the fifth century BC. Dioscorides, Paul of Aegina, Pliny, and Galen all referred to the plant, which is said to relieve excessive pain, remove the effects of shock, and have a tonic effect on the mind and body. The name St. John probably refers to John the Baptist, whom tradition said was born on the summer solstice. It was claimed that the red spots visible on the underside of some of the herb's leaves symbolized the blood of St. John, who was beheaded by Herod. In 1907 Ellingwood a famous Herbalist of the time listed the uses as for muscular bruises, deep soreness, painful parts, a sensation of throbbing in the body without fever. Burning pain, or deep soreness of the spine upon pressure, spinal irritation, and circumscribed areas of intense soreness over the spinal cord or ganglia. Concussional shock or injury to the spine, lacerated or punctured wounds in any location, accompanied with great pain. In the times of horse and carriages Homoeopaths were using it on horses to prevent tetanus after injuries to the hoofs mainly from puncture wounds there from nails or similar objects as these wounds on the hoof were prone to tetanus. Hypericum has been one of the main Homoeopathic First Aid Remedies for hundreds of years used alone or mixed with Calendula in a solution called HYPERCAL. After the 1930's it faded from popularity, but was used by the Russians in WW2 as a replacement for morphine in Lotion and Potencies

Dose - 1 to 4mls 3 times a day.

Hops
Humulus lupulus

Actions - Sedative, hypnotic, bitter, antiseptic, visceral antispasmodic, astringent, nervine.

Famed for its tonic and nervine properties, pain reliever, sleep inducer, antiseptic, tension that leads to restlessness, headache, indigestion, mucous colitis. Good for when digestive problems are caused by worry or nerves. One of the main remedies for IBS. Acts on the central nervous system and calms and eases anxiety. **Doses** - Tincture 1 to 4mls 3 times daily, 1 teaspoon of dried flowers in tea 3 times a day or just before bed. **Caution** - Do not use in depression.

Lemon Balm
Melissa Officinalis

Actions - Nervous system tonic and relaxant, antispasmodic, carminative, sedative, diaphoretic, frebrifuge, antidepressant, anti-viral, anti-microbial, anti-thyroid, choleretic, mild analgesic, antispasmodic, anti-histamine, hepatic, cardio-tonic and used for hypertension.

Specific use for dyspepsia associated with anxiety or a depressive mood. For digestive relief Lemon Balm is best consumed as a tea taken immediately after meals and also helps the liver and gallbladder. Lemon Balm contains rosmarinic acid an enzyme which increases GABA (gamma amino-butyric acid) in the brain which is one of the inhibitory neurotransmitters used by the brain to prevent over-excitement and attain balance. Increased stimulation of GABA receptors produces a sedative or calming effect which is why it is used as an anti-anxiety herb. This herb combines well with Valerian especially in helping with sleep. Indicated in hyperthyroidism (inhibits TSH (thyroid-stimulating hormone) binding to receptors), anxiety, restlessness, palpitations, headache, and excitability and also is a mild anti-depressant. Can be used for hypertension. Strengthens the brain and its resistance to stress and shock, and lifts the spirits. It has tonic effects on the heart and circulatory system. Can be used topically for gout and internally for rheumatism and neuralgias. Historically Melissa also known as Lemon Balm and was believed to sharpen memory. Lemon balm can also temporarily improve cognitive decline as well as improve the mood for Alzheimer's patients. Another study addressing the use of lemon balm for Alzheimer's concluded that Melissa is one of several plants that may be useful in the prevention and treatment of Alzheimer's disease due to its ability to inhibit acetylcholinesterase and its antioxidant activity. Said to improve cognitive function and reduce agitation in patients. Use this herb for a few months and then take a break for a month and see what happens and make a judgement from that. **Precautions** - Lemon Balm should not be used during pregnancy or lactation. Due to its anti-thyroid action it should not be taken by people with thyroid conditions. Do not take with mental health drugs without advice from a doctor or pharmacist. If you take it when you are sleepy do not drive. **Parts Used** – Aerial. **Dose** – Tincture 2 to 6mls 3 times a day. **Infusion** - 2 to 3 teaspoonful's infused for 10 minutes 3 times daily or when needed.

Lime Flower
Tilia europea

Actions - Nervine, antispasmodic, hypotensive, diaphoretic, diuretic, sedative, mild astringent, anti-inflammatory, peripheral vasodilator, anti-coagulant.

Possesses powerful nerve and blood cleansing properties, used for fits and nervous twitching of all kinds including epilepsy, nervous tension, as a prophylactic against arteriosclerosis, migraines, feverish colds and flu. It is hypotensive; although it is rarely strong enough on its own to reduce blood pressure, it will reduce hypertension when associated with arteriosclerosis and nervous tension. Indicated in hysterical states, headaches, palpitations and nervous dyspepsia. Also notable as a diaphoretic (reduces fevers) and is often used in colds and flu. **Heart Health** - Used for atherosclerosis when the arteries lose their flexibility and elasticity which is the main cause of heart disease. Linden helps to maintain the smooth inner surface and elasticity of the blood vessel walls. One of the active ingredients in Linden is an essential oil called farnesol which acts as a sedative helping to relax the cardiovascular system which in turn helps to curb stress and anxiety. **Respiratory System** - The main uses of Lime Flowers in the past was to treat coughs, colds and the flu. It contains mucilage which soothes the irritated membranes of the throat and it is known to decrease mucus production. Lime Flowers are rich in antioxidant flavonoids and anti-inflammatory compounds that can help to reduce cold and flu symptoms such as inflamed membranes in the respiratory tract. Being a diaphoretic it can help if a cold or the flu turns into a fever by inducing a bout of sweating which can often break the fever. **Digestion** - Acts as a carminative herb and bitter tonic that can be used to aid a digestive upset especially in the tea form. Can stimulate digestion while reducing gastrointestinal discomfort. Linden tea can be especially useful for excessive gas causing the stomach to push up and put pressure on the heart. The anti-spasmodic action of Lime Flowers works by relieving spasms in the intestinal tract. **Uses** - Treatment of all nervous ailments especially epilepsy, twitching, vertigo, good for colds and to remove mucous from the system, treatment of vomiting, heart pains, fevers and the treatment of tumors by poultice.

Dose - 1 to 2mls of tincture 3 times a day. Tea, 1 teaspoon full infused in a cup 3 to 5 times a day.

Licorice
Glycyrrhiza glabra

Actions - Anti bacterial, anti-viral, expectorant, demulcent, anti-inflammatory, adrenal tonic, anti-spasmodic, mild laxative, nutritive. Licorice improves macrophage activity and increases the production of interferon which is antiviral. Licorice extract also has broad spectrum anti-microbial effects along with being an antioxidant protecting the tissues especially those of the liver from free radical damage. The root part is used , licorice is one of our best demulcents especially for sore throats and painful and inflamed airways where it hurts to cough and is also good for gastric ulcers as it coats and soothes them giving them protection and reducing the inflammation, it is also nutritive and slightly laxative, It contains the building blocks of hormones, has a marked effect on the endocrine system and the glands of the body, catarrh, bronchitis, coughs, gastric and peptic ulcers, abdominal colic. Can be used for treating inflammatory and allergic conditions. A recent study at the Institute of Medical Microbiology and Virology, Kiel, Germany, researchers found that licorice extract produced a potent effect against strains of H. pylori which are the main culprits for Peptic Ulcers.

Uses - Treatment of cough, inflamed throat, pneumonia, pleurisy, TB, all catarrhal conditions, gallstones, chronic constipation, arthritis, fatigue, female infertility, pains of colic, stress, easing gastric ulcers, inhibits the herpes simplex virus.

Dose - 1 to 3mls of the tincture 3 times a day.

Caution - Do not use with high blood pressure. Long term use can also raise the blood pressure.

Mistletoe
Viscum album

Actions - Cardiac tonic, hypotensive, diuretic, antispasmodic, peripheral dilator, cardiac depressant, blood pressure normalizer, sedative, antitumor, anti-inflammatory, immune enhancer, has nervine properties on vascular system. **Uses** - Specific for arterial hypertension, arteriolosclerosis, nervous tachycardia, hypertensive headaches, hypertrophy of the heart with valvular insufficiency, dropsy of the extremities, weak pulse and labored breathing, has a wide application for treating nervous diseases, reduces bleeding. The Herbalist David Hoffman says *"Mistletoe opens up circulation to areas that have been cut off from adequate blood supply by tension. It reduces cardiovascular tension and blood pressure, while bringing in new blood, blood sugar, and healing to areas long cut off, tensed up, weakened, or damaged."* Reduces the symptoms of high blood pressure, particularly headaches and dizziness. Good for anxiety and panic attack as

Mistletoe acts to lower the stress hormone cortisol, bringing the nerves down to a more manageable level. Improves concentration, insomnia, tinnitus and epilepsy. Soothes and tones the nervous system, acts directly on the vagus nerve to reduce heart rate whilst strengthening the wall of the peripheral capillaries. Useful for nervous tachycardia and headaches from high blood pressure. Mistletoe has been used traditionally as a relaxant and herbal remedy for sleep for centuries. Mistletoe is also now being considered immune stimulant which can stimulate and modulate the immune system. **Precautions** – Pregnancy and not for children. May clash with some medications. **Combinations** - Combines well with Hawthorn Berries and Lime Blossom in the treatment of high blood pressure. **Contra Indications** - Berries are toxic. **Dose** – 1 to 3mls of tincture 3 times daily. Infusion 1 to 2 teaspoon full to cup of boiling water.

Motherwort
Leonurus cardiaca

Actions - Sedative, emmenagogue, antispasmodic, cardiac tonic. nervine, nervous system tonic, antibacterial, anti-fungal, hypothryoid, diaphoretic, cardiotonic, anti-arrhythmic, vasoconstrictor, circulatory stimulant, hypotensive, hepatic, laxative, antispasmodic, mild uterine stimulant.

As its species name indicates, it has long been considered a nerve and heart remedy. It strengthens heart function, particularly where it is weak. Antispasmodic and sedative, the herb causes relaxation rather than drowsiness. Motherwort is considered a life giving plant, beneficial for all female disorders and a general heart tonic, specific for over rapid heartbeat brought on by anxiety or tension, lowers high blood pressure and is used for the pains of birth and given for a few days after so as to prevent bleeding and infection. Indicated in nervous debility with irritation and unrest. The hypotensive action is due to its vasodilatory effect, which also serves to increase circulation to the reproductive organs. A specific for cardiac disorders of nervous origin such as tachycardia secondary to anxiety. Will also promote blood flow to female reproductive organs and balances hormones affecting the menstrual cycle as well as hyperthyroidism. **Heart Health** - As a mild vasodilator and anti-spasmodic motherwort relaxes smooth muscles, one of those muscles being the heart. Its calming nature has also been shown to slow heart palpitations and a rapid heartbeat, making it an excellent remedy for cardiac anxiety. Helps regulate uneven heart beats especially when caused by stress and anxiety. Can help to decrease cholesterol and triglycerides preventing blood clots and blood platelet aggregation and also slows down heart rate and decreases blood pressure and improves the heart circulation. Indicated for grief, anger and upsets. **Menstruation** - As an emmenogogue, Motherwort acts as a uterine tonic which helps to regulate menstruation, bring on delayed periods and can reduce smooth muscle cramping, especially menstrual cramps. Can be a useful tonic for menopausal changes. **Part used** - Aerial parts. **Contraindicated** – Pregnancy and menorrhagia. **Dose** - 1 to 4mls of tincture 3 times daily. Infusion - 1 teaspoonful infused to cup if water, 1 to 3 cups a day.

Passion Flower
Passiflora incarnata

Actions - Sedative, antispasmodic, anodyne, relaxant, epilepsy, shingles, asthma, hypotensive.

A good herb for insomnia and a very effective herb for nerve pains especially in conditions like shingles. This herbs focus is more on restlessness and irritability, hysteria and anxiety and is soothing to the mentally worried and overworked it acts on nervousness especially due to unrest, agitation, worry, exhaustion and cerebral excitement. Used in the treatment of convulsions, epilepsy, tremors, hypertension, nervous breakdowns, migraines and neuralgias.

Doses - Tincture 1 to 4mls 3 times daily, 1 teaspoon of dried herb in tea 3 times daily.

Skullcap
Scutellaria laterifolia

Action - Sedative, anti convulsive, tonic, nervine, antispasmodic, anodyne, hypotensive and anticonvulsant, stress, anxiety, PMS, anti depressive, alterative.

Skullcap has a wide range of use mostly focusing on the nerves and is a nervous system relaxant and tonic. Relaxes nervous tension while helping to strengthen the central nervous system and can be used for a wide range of conditions. Good for long term exhaustion and nervous tension. Has a specific use in the treatment of seizures and hysterical states along with epilepsy, muscular twitching, tremors and neuralgias. Used for all exhausted states and depressed conditions. Good for easing premenstrual and painful menstruation conditions due to its sedative and antispasmodic action. Use for weakness of the heart, irregular cardiac action, nervous irritation and physical exhaustion and insomnia. Skullcap eases the symptoms of drug and alcohol withdrawal such as muscle aches, shakiness, twitches, digestive distress, agitation, and poor quality sleep. Once the crisis is over Skullcap can decrease cravings for addictive substances. **Part used** - Aerial parts. **Precautions** - Avoid with tranquilisers or sedatives as Skullcap is a sedative in its own right and probably more balanced. **Combinations -** It combines well with Valerian. **Dosage-** Tincture 2 to 4mls 3 times daily. Infusion 1 to 2 teaspoons full of dried herb infused for 10 minutes.

Schisandra

Actions – Adaptogen, immune stimulant, anti-inflammatory, liver and kidney tonic, restorative, nervous system tonic, mild anti-depressant, anti-anxiety and anti-stress, adrenal tonic, antioxidant, astringent, anti-tussive, lung tonic, regulates blood pressure, anti-cholesterol, sedative.

 Of great use as a general liver protector that works well in the treatment of hepatitis. It is a liver detoxifier and works to deactivate free radicals that attack liver cells. Being extremely high in powerful antioxidants Schisandra helps to fight against free radical damage, thus lowering inflammatory responses. Can help in the nervous system by increasing the nervous reflex response and can also help in anxiety, depression, neurosis and stress. Promotes vitality and increases memory along with cognitive functions while providing resistance to stress. Is a powerful anti-anxiety herb lowering stress levels and enhancing mental performance. Because of its adaptogenic qualities it specifically reduces both mental and physical stress, exerting a normalising effect on the whole body. Schisandra reduces cortisol levels in the body (the stress hormone) and is effective in controlling changes in serotonin and adrenaline caused by stress. The herb is also considered a lung tonic because it helps the body to better utilize oxygen. Because Schisandra is high in powerful antioxidants it lowers the inflammatory responses, which in turn positively affects, tones and strengthens the immune system along with increasing physical performance and endurance and promotes recovery after surgery. Schisandra has long been used in the traditional medicines of China and Russia for a wide variety of ailments. As far back as 2697 BCE Schisandra was listed in the Yellow Emperor's Study of Inner Medicine, an encyclopedia of healing plants. **Precautions** - Mild side effects may include indigestion, nausea, headaches and skin rash. Schisandra may promote contractions of the uterine muscles and thus should not be used by pregnant women. **Contraindications** - Avoid in fever. **Part Used -** Fruit (berries). **Dose –** Tincture 3 mls up to 3 times daily. Infusions - 1 to 2 tea spoons full to cup of boiling water 3 up to 3 times daily. Can also be found in powder and tablet form.

St John's Wort

Hypericum

Medicinal Actions - Anti-inflammatory, astringent, anti-viral, anti-spasmodic, nervine, vulnerary, antibacterial and antidepressant. St John's Wort is perhaps the most studied herb for depresion with literally thousands of studies and clinical trials performed to assess its usefulness as an antidepressant. Many studies have found the herb to be equally as effective as traditional antidepressants, but with fewer side effects in mild to moderately depressed patients. This is not meant to be used in major suicidal depression. Taken internally it has a sedative and pain reducing effect, which gives it a place in the treatment of neuralgia, anxiety, tension and general depression. Hyperforin which is a component of Hypericum can inhibit synaptosomal reuptake of serotonin, norepinephrine, and dopamine. It may take 2 to 4 weeks to notice clinical results when taken for depression. Useful in mild to moderate depression, anxiety, neuralgia and myalgia's and generally for pains shooting down nerve pathways. This herb is antiviral both internally and topically. **Contraindications** - Speeds up the elimination of many and can interfere with MAOIs, SSRIs, narcotics and reserpine. Do not use St. John's Wort during pregnancy or lactation. **Caution** - Photosensitivity can occur in susceptible individuals. Fair-skinned individuals should take precautions when exposed to the sun and the elderly should use protective eyewear when exposed also. **Part Used** – Aerial and flowering parts. **Dosage** – Tincture 2 to 4mls three times daily. Infusion – 1 to 2 teaspoonsful of herb infused into a cup of boiling water taken 3 times daily.

Valerian
Valeriana officinalis

Actions - Sedative, hypnotic, antispasmodic, carminative, hypotensive, anxiety, emmenagogue, PMS, anti depressive, Nervous System relaxant.

One of the most relaxing nervines available that can be used to safely reduce tension and anxiety and is also a very effective herb for chronic insomnia. Valerian root has been shown to increase GABA (Gamma-aminobutyric acid) levels in the brain which can in turn not only reduce the amount of time taken to fall asleep but can also improve the quality of sleep too.

As an antispasmodic it will give relief to any cramp like and colicky pains and is a good pain reliever in general helping with rheumatic and migraine pains. The essential oil can help in the relief of pain especially if rubbed (diluted) on to the skin for rheumatic conditions or as added to part of a formula. As a pain reliever it is most indicated where that pain is associated with tension such as muscle problems and migraines. Has a powerful muscle relaxing effect on smooth and skeletal muscles and can be helpful in easing menstrual cramps. It can effectively calm the severe uterine muscle contractions experienced by some women during menstruation. GABA also helps to calm anxiety along with valerenic acid and valerenol and also hels in keeping stress levels down and helping in the control of blood pressure. **Precautions** - Not recommended during pregnancy or breast feeding. If it has been taken for a long time it can cause withdrawal symptoms if stopped abruptly. Some individuals will react paradoxically to Valerian and will actually be stimulated by it. Not recommended for those taking barbituates or benzodiazepine medication. **Parts Used** – Root. **Doses** - Tincture 2 to 4mls 3 times daily. 1 to 2 teaspoons full of root in tea 3 times daily or taken when needed.

Withania (Ashwagandha)

Actions - Adaptogen, analgesic, anti-tumor, hormone regulator, pregnancy tonic, rejuvinative, anti-inflammatory, sedative, anti-anemic.

Used to restore health to the nervous system and eases stress and mental exhaustion. Good for debility, nervous exhaustion especially due to stress and chronic diseases especially those marked by inflammation. Retards various aspects of the aging process and increases stamina. Promotes mental clarity and improves memory and stamina. Relieves pain by lowering serotonin levels which contribute to the sensitivity of pain receptors in the body. Tonic for the elderly and improves conditions associated with ageing. Promotes recovery after illness and during convalescence and has great use in various chronic diseases involving inflammation. Can aid bone degeneration, rheumatism, joint pain and neuralgias.

Dose - As on packet.

Introduction to Herbal Medicine

Herbal Medicine has been in use and developed continuously since the beginning of time. It mainly evolved from observations from what plants did and the affects they had on people along with their animals. There is also what they call the Doctrine of Signatures which works like this, that flower really looks like an eye, maybe it helps sore eyes? I'll give it a try as my eyes are so sore and red. You know my eye really feels a lot better now, I think I will call that plant Eye Bright (Euphrasia) and tell my friends all about it especially my Dad who gets sore eyes to. In this way hundreds of plants were identified that have a medical action and no doubt there were also a lot of casualties on the way. The next great leap in herbal medicine was the Roman Empire of 2000 years ago. The Great Armies of Rome all had their own Medical Corps with Doctors, Battle Surgeons and Orderlies. It was these men who already had the knowledge of the Greeks that started to put together the best medical manuals in the world while at the same time started developing and using medical instruments and tools, some of which are still used today. As the Romans conquered the known world more medicines and knowledge were found and assimilated. The next great leap was modern Chemistry which allowed us to see exactly what herbs were made up of and what parts of the herb causes its medical action. Drug companies have made billions of Dollars from this information as they find the main active ingredient and then make a synthetic version of it, one good example that we all know of is Valium which is the synthetic version of the active ingredient from the herb Valerian. Leaving aside the Drug Companies let's see how Chemistry changed the way that modern herbalists think. Modern science allows us to now know what Actions our herbs perform on the body so we shall carry on using Valerian as an example and see what Medical Actions of Valerian has on the body. The Actions of Valerian are Sedative, Hypnotic (sleep inducing), Anti Spasmodic (stops twitches, cramps etc), Hypotensive (lowers Blood Pressure) and Carminative (calms and relaxes the tummy especially if you are worried sick). Herbalists call Valerian the Herbal Tranquillizer and if you look at the actions you can see why, for if you can't sleep and your blood pressures up along with a gurgling tummy and an eye constantly twitching you definitely need to be calmed down. The modern herbalist is trained to think in actions. There are many reasons for this but the main ones are to stop them from just using a handful of their favorite herbs and to train the mind to work in the method of thinking in actions that are needed. If we start thinking in the actions that are needed for a patient it makes us consider the problem in far more depth than just using our favorite herb, and it forces our thinking to be far more holistic by taking in consideration the whole of the patient not just the part or the system we wish to treat. Let's take a look at thinking in actions. The patient has a cough, then the coughs can't stop and it sounds a bit like whooping cough. The patient also sounds a little hoarse and the temperature is also elevated. The actions that come into mind for this are expectorant for the cough, antispasmodics for the whooping quality of the cough and demulcents to sooth the sore throat. These are the obvious actions and we can add many more if we wish such as immune boosters for acute diseases, diaphoretics to reduce the temperature and prevent a fever and the list goes on but it's always best to keep it simple. Next we look at how Herbal Actions are used in making Herbal Formulas. Another point to make before we go to the formula making is that Professional Herbalists use Herbs in the form of Tinctures (water and alcohol solutions) as this allows them to mix formulas in any proportions that they like and also allows long term storage without spoiling. Along with using tinctures I also use herbs in powder form which can be a good and very cheap form to use and you can mix the powders into Herbal Formulas just as you do for tinctures but here you use capsules. If you want to use capsules you can buy capsule machines, some do 50 at a time while the ones I use do 100 at a time. I buy my empty capsules by the thousands but you could maybe start off buying 500 at a time with ebay being a good place to find them and the machines.

Making Herbal Formulas

You should never have more than 5 Herbs in a herbal formula otherwise you will start to lose track of what you are doing and how the formula is changing the symptoms. Always try to keep things simple. One of the herbs in the formula is used to force the formula into the body, to keep it simple we will only use three; they are Licorice, Ginger and Cayenne. As an example we will continue with the patient with a cough. After further study of the case we decide that this is an Acute Disease for it came on quickly and is fast acting and not slow like a Chronic Disease. Listening to the patients cough we decide that it is a dry cough and the patient has not got a runny nose. Let's list the actions to consider.

Expectorants - Licorice, Aniseed, Fennel, Garlic and Mullein

Antispasmodics - Aniseed and Fennel

Demulcents - Licorice and Coltsfoot

Immune Boosters - Echinacea

Anti-Bacterial and Virals – Garlic, Licorice and Echinacea

Out of the above I would choose Licorice, Echinacea, Garlic, Aniseed and Fennel. I would make the formula in this strength.

Formula

Licorice - 20%

Garlic - 15%

Echinacea - 15%

Aniseed - 30%

Fennel - 20%

These herbs are listed below. Read through them and consider why I used them, there are three obvious ones for Licorice alone with the first being to force the assimilation of the formula into the body. The second is for its expectorant action and third is its demulcent action in case the throat is sore and raw. Next time you see a little kid eating heaps of licorice get them to open their mouth and look at their tongue which will be going black from the Licorice along with the throat etc, and know that you are looking at the demulcent action of Licorice working by coating and soothing and whatever it coats will also be getting its anti-inflammatory action as well. The most important reason that you use the Actions Method for Herbal Prescribing is so that you can concentrate the Actions which are most needed for example, if it's a Bacterial Infection concentrate on the Anti Bacterials, if it's a Viral infection concentrate on the Anti Virals and in this case when you look at the herbs below you will see that three of them have a expectorant action. Hopefully you are now beginning to see the importance of working in actions for if you don't concentrate a large part of the battle on the causes you may have lost the battle from the start. Read through all the Actions listed in Herbal Actions in the book and then do a study in depth of at least five Actions of your choice making the first two the Anti Bacterials and Anti Virals. Start trying to train your mind into thinking in Actions.

Licorice

Actions - Expectorant, demulcent, anti-inflammatory, adrenal agent, anti-spasmodic, mild laxative. The root part is used, possessing unique pectoral and emollient properties; it is also nutritive and slightly laxative. It contains the building blocks of hormones, has a marked effect on the endocrine system, catarrh, gastric and peptic ulcers, abdominal colic. Its ability to soothe irritated mucous membranes and to break up phlegm and ease coughing sees licorice employed in respiratory conditions, coughing, bronchitis, and chest colds. Can be used for treating inflammatory and allergic conditions. Licorice has effects on the adrenal glands which are protective, restorative, tonic and stimulatory. **Uses** - Treatment of cough, inflamed throat, pneumonia, pleurisy, TB, all catarrhal conditions, gallstones, chronic constipation. **Dose** – 1 to 3mls of tincture 3 times daily. **Caution** - Do not use with high blood pressure. Long term use depletes potassium which raises the blood pressure. Don't use with steroids.

Garlic

Actions - Immune stimulant, anti-bacterial, anti-viral, anti-fungal, anti-septic, anti-oxidant, diaphoretic, cholagogue, hypotensive, anti-spasmodic, vermifuge and many more.

The plant is rich in volatile oil and sulphur and because of its remarkable penetrating, disinfecting and mucous expelling powers garlic is a valuable basic remedy for the treatment of all ailments in which the cleansing of the blood stream and expulsion of mucous accumulations is required. Garlic is one of our main herbs used to prevent and treat respiratory infections. Anyone who has had garlic breath has experienced this herb's aromatic compounds being excreted through their lungs which is why garlic's active ingredients can be so effective for respiratory complaints. Garlic is extremely effective in dissolving and cleansing cholesterol from the blood stream, it stimulates the digestive tract, kills worms, parasites and harmful bacteria, normalizes blood pressure, reduces fever, gas and cramps. I use Garlic in oil form (Garlic Oil Capsules) for respiratory infections as the oil goes into the blood stream fast and a lot of it exits via the lungs hence the garlic breath. **Uses-** All infections, coughs, colds, flu, bronchitis, all fevers, pulmonary conditions, gastric and skin complaints, rheumatism, all worms and ringworm, ticks and lice. Acts on Bacteria, Viruses and Internal Parasites. **Dose** – 3000mg Garlic Oil tabs are the best way to go as tis gets into the blood fast. For those who cannot tolerate the breath use Kyloc the Japanese aged form as this is odorless.

Echinacea

Actions - Immune stimulant, anti-microbial, anti-inflammatory, alterative, healing.

This herb is an infection fighter active against strep bacteria (abscesses and boils), a blood cleanser, (blood poisons, snake bites, poisonous insects) and a glandular and lymphatic system cleanser. Use it particularly for respiratory infections and for any disease above the waist. This is one of our main immune boosters for the acute diseases. Echinacea stimulates the bone marrow to make more white blood cells which are our main infection killers and why we only use it in short bursts. Use as a prophylactic to protect from infections especially when traveling or before going into Hospital. **Uses** - All infections, depressed immune function, inflammatory conditions, allergies, effective against both bacteria and viruses. **Dose** – 1 to 4mls of tincture. **Warning** - Do not use continually as you will burn out the immune system give a few weeks break after 3 weeks. Beware also in the use of allergies for you could be building up the immune system just to attack itself.

Aniseed

Actions - Antispasmodic, carminative, expectorant, parasiticide, antimicrobial, galactagogue.

This is a herb with many uses, some of the main uses are intestinal colic and flatulence, a good digestive tonic and appetite stimulant, a good expectorant and along with its antispasmodic action it can be used for such conditions as bronchitis and whooping cough. Aniseed has mild estrogenic effects and can be used as a good herb for relieving some of the symptoms of menopause. This herb has a reputation of increasing milk production in nursing mothers, promoting menstruation and also facilitating childbirth. It is also said to increase libido in men and women. **Doses -** Mainly used as a tea, 1 to 2 teaspoonfuls of seeds add boiling water, cover and leave for 5 to 10 minutes.

Fennel

Actions - Carminative, aromatic, anti-spasmodic, stimulant, galactagogue, expectorant.

The herb possesses highly antiseptic and tonic properties. The primary use of fennel is to relieve bloating, but it also settles stomach pain, stimulates the appetite and is diuretic and anti-inflammatory.

Uses - Gastric ailments, relieves flatulence and colic, stimulates appetite, inflammation of the bowels, acute constipation (raw roots daily), fevers, cramps, worms, indigestion, all eye ailments, bronchitis, coughs, muscular and rheumatic pains use the oil. Externally used as an eye wash to treat eye infections. **Dose** - 2 to 4mls of tincture 3 times daily.

The more you look at the formula and compare it to the herbs I chose the more you will learn and see the different reasoning that was considered but do this over time when you have learnt more about herbs and are getting used to using them.

How to Make Herbal Tinctures

Tinctures are made by steeping the Herb plant material in a mixture of alcohol and water. Alcohol is usually always used at strength of 45%. The alcohol in this mixture will extract all the essential oils from the herb while the water will extract all that is water soluble, so between the both we are getting most of the medicinal properties out of the herb. The proportions of herb to liquid are usually 1 part herb to 5 parts liquid. So find a suitable container (I use a big one liter preserving jar with a good sealing lid) and put into it 100grams of your chosen herb and to that add 500mls of our 45% solution of alcohol and water. Seal the lid and shake well for about a minute. Leave the jar on the window sill so the sun can shine on the jar for two weeks. The jar must be shaken for at least a minute every day. After 2 weeks open and filter the contents of the jar. I use a large pouring jug into which I place a funnel and then place a coffee filter in the funnel and pour the jar contents through the funnel being careful not to let too much herb spill into the filter and block it up. When you get to the bottom of the jar you can crush the herb in your fist so as to extract the last of the liquid. After this is completed you then get your chosen storage bottle, put a funnel into its neck followed by a coffee filter and then filter the jug into the bottle so it is double filtered. Next we label the bottle, put the date, name and proportions e.g. 1 to 5 also state the recommended dose. Store in a cool and dark place. Most Professional Homoeopaths and Herbalists have access to pure alcohol so for them it is fairly easy to make tinctures while for the lay person they will probably have a hard time. An alternative is to use Vodka as strong as you can find it or find a way to twist the authorities arm into giving alcohol at 45%. Don't even try to get pure alcohol as it is dangerous and can turn people blind and they won't give it to you. Or in the case of my brother get a still.

How to Make Infusions

Infusions are a bit like making a cup of tea except we don't use milk. Infusions are used for the soft parts of the herb such as the flowers, leaves and fine twigs. The proportions for infusions are 1 to 20 e.g. 1 part herb to 20 parts water. Infusions are used for the more water soluble herbs. Infusions can be made from a single herb or from a combination of herbs and may be drunk hot or cold. The water should be just off the boil before being poured on the herb and if you are making an infusion of a herb strong in essential oils such as Peppermint always cover the top of the cup to stop the essential oils from escaping in steam while the infusion is brewing. Allow up to 10 minutes to brew. It is best to make herbal teas fresh each day. You can experiment on yourself by getting Chamomile and Peppermint tea bags from the supermarket. Use honey as a sweetener.

How to Make Decoctions

Decoctions are used for the more hard woody substances of the herb such as barks, berries or roots. The process of decoction is far more vigorous then infusion as it involves heating the plant material in cold water, bringing it to the boil and simmering for 20 to 40 minutes. The finished ratio for decoctions is again 1 part herb to 20 parts water; remember to add more water at the beginning so you wind up with the 1 to 20 after steam loss. This form of preparation is no good for the herbs that are high in essential oils as these will all be lost in the steam.

How to Make Your Own Creams

Herbal Tinctures for medicating creams will be Calendula, St John's Wort (Hyrpericum), Arnica and Witch Hazel. Use Comfrey and Castor Oil as and when needed. Find a good cheap seconds shop and look for Vitamin E or Lanolin cream in a really big jar so that you can fill lots of normal sized jars. For a normal sized jar use half to three quarters of a small teaspoon full of tincture poured on top of a cream filled jar. We will do a hard one first which is the mixture of Calendula and Hypericum tinctures which are two of our best wound healers mixed together. Calendula heals and closes wounds fast (so make sure they are clean) while Hypericum is more the pain killer, antiseptic and tetanus prevention. To make this easier find a small 10 to 15ml bottle and label it Hypercal and fill it half and half of each so from now on you have a bottle of Hyercal. Next fill a normal sized jar fill of your chosen cream then bang the base of the jar fairly hard twice on the kitchen table which should settle all the cream to the bottom of the jar, if it looks as though it needs more cream repeat the process. Get a small teaspoon and three quarter fill it and pour on the cream. Next turn the teaspoon upside down and use the handle to stir the cream in the jar. After two and a half minutes of stirring you will start thinking this isn't working. After five minutes you will think there it goes. Some creams are faster than others but most take a lot of stirring. This is the way we medicate creams. When doing this get to know the herb, smell it, then put a drop on your finger and taste it. Is it really bitter? If so it will be a good digestive herb, get to know your new friends. As we age and get older the skin becomes thinner so we become prone to more injuries especially on the hands. Every year I would always give my parents a big jar of Hypercal for Christmas and at the end of the year it was usually close to the empty.

Cuts and Wounds

The first consideration is to stop the bleeding, rule out any deeper internal damage and clean and disinfect the wound. To stop the bleeding apply pressure. Calendula is one of the main lotions used for cleaning wounds as it is gentle, soothing, astringent, healing and anti-microbial so it kills the germs as well. Calendula has a tendency of sometimes welding the skin together (handy for closing knife cuts) this is more noticeable on wounds with clean cut edges. Because of this tendency it is very important to make sure that all wounds are very clean and no dirt remains inside. Now we will introduce you to Hypericum (St John's Wort), I use Hypericum lotion on wounds that are in very nerve rich areas, a good example is crush injuries to the finger as we all know how painful and sensitive a wound is to this area. As well as being used for nerve damage Hypericm is also astringent so it will help in stopping the bleeding and its anti-inflammatory action should help to reduce the swelling. I usually get a separate bottle and fill it up with half Hypericum and half Calendula tincture and call this bottle Hypercal. I use this bottle for making my lotions for deep wounds and on nervy areas. Consider also that these are both astringents so our power to stop bleeding has been increased. Tea Tree Oil is good for small wounds and has a strong antibacterial action but can sometimes hurt in open wounds. The oil is good where there is infection as it draws pus to a head. If you have a clean cut wound fairly deep but on the border line of getting stitches and have managed to stop the bleeding here's a way of putting a kind of skin graft on it which will hold the wound shut while you decide what to do but clean the wound first calendula lotion as this will sometimes seal it. Break and empty an egg. On the inside of the egg shell you will see a plastic like skin, peel this off and lay across the wound wet side down. The skin is also meant to have an antibiotic action which protects the egg. If you are going to try to get away without stitches try to immobilize the area for a couple of days so you don't accidentally rip the wound open again and use plenty of Calendula to close the wound.

Herbal Treatment

1. Deal with bleeding and clean wound under running tap water if possible.

2. Do the final cleaning with Calendula or Hypercal lotion mixed 1 to 20 parts water.

3. Cover and protect the wound if you think it is necessary.

4. When wound is dry and healing (if weeping use Hypercal lotion) you can use Calendula cream with maybe Comfrey cream as well for scar prevention or if the wound is healing slowly. You can also medicate a little bit of Calendula cream with Hypericum to make a Hypercal cream for a healing wound giving off nervy pain. Hypericum is the next most well used lotion, its main calling is for wounds of the very nervy parts of the body such as the fingers, tail bone, lips or for any part that really hurts and is nervy. One of the leading symptoms for Hypericum is shooting pains along the nerve pathways from the injured area. Hypericum is good for infections and septic conditions in nervy areas and I would use it with Calendula for any infection in a wound especially deep wounds. In the past Hypericum was used to prevent Tetanus in deep puncture wounds especially from rusty metal objects. Remember infections are trying to get the rubbish out of the body so when they begin to discharge do not try to stop the discharge let the body get rid of its rubbish.

Hypercal - Which is a half and half mixture of Hypericum and Calendula tinctures, you can use this to make lotions when you want the effects of both Calendula and Hypericum together. An example would be an infected crushed finger.

Creams- Calendula and Hypericum creams can be used when the healing begins and are applied for the same reasons as the lotions but always remember the lotion gets in better. Creams are more for the latter stages of healing.

Our Two Main Wound Herbs
Calendula

Medicinal Actions- Anti-inflammatory, astringent, vulnerary, anti-fungal, germicide, demulcent. **Part Used** - The Flowers. **Used For.-**.Minor skin problems, cuts, abrasions, rashes, spots, acne, slow healing wounds, skin ulcers and to improve post-operative healing, fungal skin infections such as thrush, athletes foot and ring worm. Used to stop bleeding, heal bruises and sprains, skin ulcers, minor burns and scolds, healing, soothing, and anti-microbial. As a douche or bath to treat vaginal thrush. Gargle for sore throat and tonsillitis. It can be applied as a lotion, ointment, wash, gargle, compress, poultice, bath and douche as required. Use as a lotion (1 to 20) to clean wounds, one of our main germicides for wounds and if Hypericum is added to the lotion you may prevent tetanus as well. **Caution** - Calendula closes wounds rapidly so make sure they are very clean and no foreign bodies remain. **How To Use**– For a very serious wound bleeding medicate a cloth with tincture and apply with pressure to the area till bleeding stops. Use as a Lotion one part tincture to twenty parts water to wash out wounds or medicate affected area, make at 1 to 10 for bleeding or fungal infections. Use a teaspoon of tincture to medicate a small jar of cream then stir rapidly for 5 minutes or less if it mixes in fast, usually they don't. I usually get a cheap Vitamin E cream from one of the big cheap wholesalers and medicate the cream with Calendula. Use Tincture for medicating creams. **Herbal Actions of Calendula - Germicide** - Calendula is a strong antiseptic, due to it wide variety of chemical constituents, including carotenoids which speed up wound healing and strengthens cells. Along with fighting bacteria in topical preparations, Calendula also fights viruses and fungi, particularly those on the skin and nails. **Anti-inflammatory**- Where-ever there is skin irritation and redness, an anti-inflammatory action is needed to help the skin recover. With Calendula also being a Germicide it takes out the cause of the inflammation which is usually infection. Here the triterpenealcohols in Calendula exert their powerful inflammation reducing effects. They contribute to the plants overall ability to heal wounds such as burns, cuts and grazes as effectively or more effectively than conventional steroidal applications. **Astringent** - The most important use of the astringents in First Aid is to stop the bleeding and they do this by causing the arterioles and arteries to spasm at the cut end. Calendula is well known for stopping bleeding especially in the hard to stop areas such as the palms of hands where in the serious cases tinctures can be used on cloth and put in the palm and the patient made to make a fist. Calendulas astringent action can be used to improve blood vessels and tone and tighten up skin cells, thus reducing the occurrence of complaints such as hemorrhoids. (Use with Witchazel and Hypericum). Many new mums find themselves looking for a natural way to combat this condition and it is important to do so as there is a risk of developing blood clots. **Demulcent**- The soothing properties of Calendula are due to many of its chemical constituents in particular the triterpene saponins and mucilage. Both of these substances provide a soft and soothing healing effect on external skin surfaces.

Hops
Humulus lupulus

Actions - Sedative, hypnotic, bitter, antiseptic, visceral antispasmodic, astringent, nervine.

Famed for its tonic and nervine properties, pain reliever, sleep inducer, antiseptic, tension that leads to restlessness, headache, indigestion, mucous colitis. Good for when digestive problems are caused by worry or nerves. One of the main remedies for IBS. Acts on the central nervous system and calms and eases anxiety. **Digestive System** – Nervous digestive conditions with insufficient secretions and over excitability of the nervous system. Visceral smooth muscle tensions affecting digestive and bowel functions, mucous colitis, spastic constipation, nervous dyspepsia, mucous colitis with Chamomile. Reduced stomach acidity, check fermentation. **Nervous System** – Sedative to encourage restful sleep, insomnia due to worry or nervous debility with Valerian, reduces symptoms of nervous tension, nerve pains, excitability and hysteria with Valerian. **Doses** - Tincture 1 to 4mls 3 times daily, 1 teaspoon of dried flowers in tea 3 times a day or just before bed. **Caution** - Do not use in depression.

Hypericum - (St John's Wort)

Medicinal Actions- Anti-inflammatory, astringent, anti-viral, anti-spasmodic, nervine, vulnerary, antibacterial. **Part Used** - Aerial parts. **Uses** –For First Aid we are concentrating on external use only. Used for wounds with pains that shoot along the nerves in nerve rich areas such as the fingers, lips, tail bone and toes. As a lotion it will speed the healing of wounds and bruises and is used where there is nerve damage and the possibility of tetanus. The main remedy for puncture wounds as it can sometimes kill tetanus. Good for varicose veins especially the painful kind and mild burns. Patients recovering from surgery where the nerves have been damaged often recover faster with Hypericum. For inflamed joints and rheumatic pain, painful abscesses, bad insect stings, damaged nerves from impact injuries, sprains and ulcers. Eases the pain in conditions such as lumbago, sciatica and Shingles (antiviral) where a cream can be used on the sore and the oil applied along the affected nerve path. As a lotion it is commonly mixed with Calendula, Homoeopaths call this lotion Hypercal. **How To Use** - Use as a Lotion one part tincture to twenty parts water to wash out wounds or medicate affected area, make at 1 to 10 for painful and dirty wounds. Mix with Calendula in large painful bleeding wounds with a chance of tetanus. Use Tincture for medicating creams. In **1907 Ellingwood** a famous Herbalist of the time listed the uses for muscular bruises, deep soreness, painful parts, and a sensation of throbbing in the body without fever. Burning pain or deep soreness of the spine upon pressure, spinal irritation and circumscribed areas of intense soreness over the spinal cord or ganglia. Concussion shock or injury to the spine, lacerated or punctured wounds in any location, accompanied with great pain. In the times of horse and carriages Homoeopaths were using it on horses to prevent tetanus after injuries to the hoofs mainly from puncture wounds from nails or similar objects as these wounds on the hoof were prone to tetanus. Hypericum has been one of the main Homoeopathic First Aid Remedies for hundreds of years used alone or mixed with Calendula in a solution called HYPERCAL. After the 1930's it faded from popularity but was used by the Russians in WW2 as a replacement for morphine in Lotion and Potencies. **Hypercal** -

Hypercal is a 50 50 mixture of Hypericum and Calendula Tinctures. This is a combination of two of the best wound healing herbs mixed together. Calendula is more for dealing with the blood vessels and bleeding along with the rapid closure of the wound so care must be taken to ensure the wound is clean and no foreign bodies are there to be sealed in. Hypericums work is more on the damaged nerves and pain as well as infections in and of the nervous system especially those caused by deep and painful puncture wounds which could harbor tetanus if not properly cleaned and dealt with. By using these two herbs together you are doubling their main actions of anti-inflammatory and astringents with the last action being good for stopping bleeding and also infection. Wounds calling for Hypercal are usually bloody and painful. Works well on long and extensive grazes and cleaning gravel rash and wounds but is mainly called for impact injuries to the lips, fingers or toes. Ideal for closing clean incisions fast and after surgical operations. So the leading symptoms for Hypercal are painful wounds. Use as a lotion at one part to ten or 1 to 20 depending on your judgment of pain and infection. In emergency bleeding use the tincture as this will spasm the arterioles but be aware that the high alcohol content will cause pain in its raw state. Use Tincture for medicating creams.

Burns

The usual rule is to place the burnt area under cold water as soon as possible. I usually leave it under there till it's nearly numb from the cold. The point to remember here is that when you take let's say your hand away from whatever burnt it the heat from the burn is still traveling inward and will continue to do so for about 15 seconds so this is why you must get to the cold water fast so you can reduce the severity and the depth of the burn. For minor burns and scolds Aloe Vera gel straight from the plants leaf can give quick relief and speed up the healing. In Herbal Medicine we use astringents for burns (with the exception being for burns that cover a very large area) as the tannins in the herbs will seal and protect the burned surface. Tannins also have a antibacterial action so this should help in the prevention of infections. Deep burns always require prompt medical attention. **Herbal Treatment - Aloe Vera** - apply to burn straight from the plant. **Witch Hazel** - Use as a lotion at about 1 to 20 strength and apply to the burn, this herb is a strong astringent and should seal and protect the surface. **Hypericum** - This can be added to the above lotion as it has some similar actions but for burns we are mainly using it to reduce the pain. Once the healing has begun you can continue applying **Aloe Vera** especially if there is still pain. Another good herb for around the edges of the burn as it heals is **Calendula Cream**.

Understanding Homoeopathy

Homoeopathy has been around now for hundreds of years and unlike most other forms of medicine its rules have not changed and will not for they are an essential truth. The main rule is Like cures Like or if we break down the word Homoeopathy homo means the same and pathy means disease. As Homoeopathy is a very hard science to learn and as it kind of sits or balances on the boarder of hard science and metaphysics I will not try to explain to you in detail what it is here as it would probably take a whole book to do this but I will say this, in the UK and a lot of countries in Europe and especially in India it is on and paid for by the National Health Systems and anything that can get a politician to open their purse must have a lot of truth in it. It is said that Homoeopathy sits on a three legged stool. What this means is that if a remedy has at least three symptoms in the same strength as your patients symptoms, then that remedy is a potential cure for their condition or if not cure it will offer relief. The more symptoms you can match to the remedy the better the remedy will work for the rule is likes cure likes not vaguely similar cures. Listed below is an example of a Homoeopathic remedy from William Boerickes Materia Medica and some of the symptoms it covers. The idea is to find one remedy that covers most of your symptoms. Pay special notice of the Mental symptoms as these are some of the most important symptoms to try to match. Notice the way it set out, the italic writing says that these symptoms are strong in the remedy. This is a very common remedy in Homoeopathy and is known as one of the Polycrests, you will see it in many of the diseases so come back here to refer to it. Relating to Dementia we can see two good symptoms in the **Mind** area with the first being Hallucinations and the next, Sensitive to disorder and confusion. Look down towards the end at **Modalities**, these tell you what makes the condition better or worse.

Arsenicum Album

A profoundly acting remedy on every organ and tissue. Its clear-cut characteristic symptoms and correspondence too many severe types of disease make its homeopathic employment constant and certain. Its general symptoms often alone lead to its successful application. Among these the all-prevailing debility, exhaustion, and *restlessness*, with *nightly aggravation*, are most important. *Great exhaustion after the slightest exertion*. This, with the peculiar irritability of fiber, gives the characteristic *irritable weakness. Burning pains*. Unquenchable thirst. Burning relieved by heat. *Seaside complaints* (*Nat mur; Aqua Marina*). Injurious effects of fruits, especially more watery ones. Gives quiet and ease to the last moments of life when given in high potency. *Fear fright and worry*. Green discharges. Infantile Kala-azar (Dr. Neatby). *Ars* should be thought of in ailments from alcoholism, *ptomaine poisoning*, stings, dissecting wounds, chewing tobacco; ill effects from decayed food or animal matter; odor of discharges is *putrid*; in complaints that return annually. Anemia and chlorosis. Degenerative changes. Gradual loss of weight from impaired nutrition. Reduces the refractive index of blood serum (also *China* and *Ferr phos*). Maintains the system under the stress of malignancy regardless of location. Malarial cachexia. *Septic infections and low vitality*.

Mind - *Great anguish and restlessness. Changes place continually. Fears*, of death, of being left alone. Great fear, with cold sweat. Thinks it useless to take medicine. Suicidal. Hallucinations of smell and sight. Despair drives him from place to place. Miserly, malicious, selfish, lacks courage. General sensibility increased (*Hep*). Sensitive to disorder and confusion.

Head - Headaches relieves by cold, other symptoms worse. Periodical burning pains, with *restlessness*; with cold skin. Hemicrania, with icy feeling of scalp and great weakness. Sensitive head in open air. Delirium tremens; cursing and raving; vicious. Head is in constant motion. Scalp *itches* intolerably; circular patches of bare spots; rough, dirty, sensitive, and covered with dry scales; nightly burning and itching; dandruff. Scalp very sensitive; cannot brush hair.

Eyes - *Burning in eyes, with acrid lachrymation.* Lids red, ulcerated, scabby, scaly, granulated. Edema *around* eyes. External inflammation, with extreme painfulness; *burning, hot,* and excoriating lachrymation. Corneal ulceration. *Intense photophobia;* better external warmth. Ciliary neuralgia, with fine burning pain.

Ears - Skin within, raw and burning. *Thin, excoriating, offensive* otorrhœa. Roaring in ears, during a paroxysm of pain.

Nose - *Thin, watery, excoriating* discharge. Nose feels *stopped up.* Sneezing *without* relief. Hay-fever and coryza; worse in open air; better indoors. *Burning* and bleeding. Acne of nose. Lupus.

Face - Swollen, pale, yellow, *cachectic,* sunken, cold, and covered with sweat (*Acetic acid*). Expression of agony. Tearing *needle-like* pains; burning. Lips black, livid. Angry, circumscribed flush of cheeks.

Mouth - Unhealthy, easily-bleeding gums. Ulceration of mouth with dryness and burning heat. Epithelioma of lips. Tongue dry, clean, and red; stitching and burning pain in tongue, ulcerated with blue color. Bloody saliva. Neuralgia of teeth; feel long and very sore; worse after midnight; better warmth. Metallic taste. *Gulping up of burning water.*

Throat - Swollen, edematous, constricted, *burning,* unable to swallow. Diphtheritic membrane, looks dry and wrinkled.

Stomach - *Cannot bear the sight or smell of food. Great thirst; drinks much, but little at a time.* Nausea, retching, vomiting, after eating or drinking. Anxiety in pit of stomach. *Burning pain.* Craves acids and coffee. Heartburn; gulping up of acid and bitter substances which seem to excoriate the throat. Long-lasting eructation's. Vomiting of blood, bile, green mucus, or brown-black mixed with blood. Stomach extremely irritable; seems raw, as if torn. Gastralgia from slightest food or drink. Dyspepsia from vinegar, acids, ice-cream, ice-water, tobacco. Terrible fear and dyspnœa, with gastralgia; also faintness, icy coldness, great exhaustion. Malignant symptoms. Everything swallowed seems to lodge in the œsophagus, which seems as if closed and nothing would pass. *Ill effects of vegetable diet, melons, and watery fruits generally*. Craves milk.

Abdomen - Gnawing, burning pains like coals of fire; relieved by heat. *Liver and spleen enlarged and painful*. Ascites and anasarca. Abdomen swollen and painful. Pain as from a wound in abdomen on coughing.

Rectum - Painful, spasmodic protrusion of rectum. Tenesmus. *Burning* pain and pressure in rectum and anus.

Stool - *Small, offensive, dark, with much prostration. Worse at night, and after eating and drinking*; from chilling stomach, alcoholic abuse, spoiled meat. Dysentery dark, bloody, very offensive. Cholera, with intense agony, prostration, and burning thirst. Body cold as ice (*Verat*). Hæmorrhoids burn like fire; relieved by heat. Skin excoriated about anus.

Urine - Scanty, burning, involuntary. Bladder as if paralysed. *Albuminous*. Epithelial cells; cylindrical clots of fibrin and globules of pus and blood. After urinating, feeling of weakness in abdomen. Bright's disease. Diabetes.

Female - Menses too profuse and too soon. Burning in ovarian region. Leucorrhœa, acrid, burning, offensive, thin. Pain as from red-hot wires; worse least exertion; causes great fatigue; better in warm room. *Menorrhagia*. Stitching pain in pelvis extending down the thigh.

Respiratory - Unable to lie down; fears suffocation. Air-passages constricted. Asthma worse midnight. Burning in chest. Suffocative catarrh. Cough worse after midnight; worse lying on back. Expectoration *scanty, frothy. Darting pain through upper third of right lung.* Wheezing respiration. Hæmoptysis with pain between shoulders; burning heat all over. Cough dry, as from sulphur fumes; *after drinking.*

Heart - Palpitation, pain, dyspnœa, faintness. Irritable heart in smokers and tobacco-chewers. *Pulse more rapid in morning* (*Sulph*). Dilatation. Cyanosis. Fatty degeneration. Angina pectoris, with pain in neck and occiput.

Back - Weakness in small of back. Drawing in of shoulders. Pain and burning in back (*Oxal ac*).

Extremities - Trembling, twitching, spasms, weakness, heaviness, uneasiness. Cramps in calves. Swelling of feet. Sciatica. Burning pains. Peripheral neuritis. Diabetic gangrene. Ulcers on heel (*Cepa; Lamium*). Paralysis of lower limbs with atrophy.

Skin - Itching, burning, swellings; œdema, eruption, papular, *dry, rough, scaly; worse cold* and scratching. Malignant pustules. Ulcers with offensive discharge. Anthrax. Poisoned wounds. Urticaria, with burning and restlessness. *Psoriasis.* Scirrhus. Icy coldness of body. Epithelioma of the skin. Gangrenous inflammations.

Sleep - Disturbed, anxious, restless. Must have head raised by pillows. Suffocative fits during sleep. Sleeps with hands over head. Dreams are full of care and fear. Drowsy, sleeping sickness.

Fever - High temperature. *Periodicity marked with adynamia.* Septic fevers. *Intermittent. Paroxysms incomplete, with marked exhaustion. Hay-fever.* Cold sweats. Typhoid, not too early; often after Rhus. Complete exhaustion. Delirium; worse after midnight. Great restlessness. Great heat about 3 am.

Modalities - *Worse,* wet weather, after midnight; from cold, cold drinks, or food. Seashore. Right side. *Better* from heat; from head elevated; warm drinks.

Complementary: *Rhus; Carbo; Phos. Thuja; Secale.* Antidotal to lead poison.

Antidotes: *Opium; Carbo; China; Hepar; Nux.* Chemical Antidotes: Charcoal; Hydrated Peroxide of Iron; Lime Water.

Compare: *Arsenic stibatum* 3x (Chest inflammations · of children, restlessness with thirst and prostration, loose mucous cough, oppression, hurried respiration, crepitant rales). *Cenchris contortrix; Iod; Phosph; China; Verat alb; Carbo; Kali phos. Epilobium* (intractable diarrhœa of typhoid). *Hoang Nan. Atoxyl.* Sodium arseniate 3x, sleeping sickness; commencing optic atrophy. *Levico Water--* (containing Ars, Iron and Copper of South Tyrol). Chronic and dyscratic skin diseases, chorea minor and spasms in scrofulous and anæmic children. Favors assimilation and increases nutrition. Debility and skin diseases, especially after the use of higher potencies where progress seems suspended. Dose. Ten drops in wine glass of warm water 3 times a day after meals (Burnett). *Sarcolatic acid* (influenza with violent vomiting).

Dose - Third to thirtieth potency. The very highest potencies often yield brilliant results.

Low attenuations in gastric, intestinal, and kidney diseases; higher in neuralgias, nervous diseases, and skin. But if only surface conditions call for it, give the lowest potencies, 2x to 3x trit. Repeated doses advisable.

Boerickes Materia Medica is the best one for use by the lay person; once you have mastered it you can move on to the many others. To make the remedies as closer a match we can we ask lots of questions like the ones below and after we gather all the answers we have what is called a good Symptom Picture which we then try to match as accurately as we can to a Remedy. Homoeopathic Repertories are used for matching symptoms to remedies but in this book you get the specific for each disease so try to match them as best as you can.

Symptom Guide Questions

1. Is there a sudden onset, what time?

2. What time of the day does the patient feel either better or worse?

3. What is the effect of motion? Jarring, walking, running?

4. What is the effect of drinking fluids? Prefers warm or cold drinks?

5. Is the patient thirsty or not at all? Sips or gulps?

6. Is the onset from exertion, overeating, weather changes, emotions?

7. Mental and emotional state of patient? This is most important.

8. Better warm room, warm air?

9. Better cool room, cool open air?

10. Respirations - dry or wet?

11. Expectoration - watery or stringy mucous, easy or difficult.

12. Is there coughing

13. Position - better or worse from sitting, standing, lying, lying on which side?

One of the main rules of Homoeopathy is the closer the match of the remedy the higher the Potency you use. Potency is a measure of strength and most of the remedies we will use will be in the 30th Potency until we get some experience, an example of how you would write this is **Pulsatilla 30C.** (don't forget the C on the end).

Remember as mentioned before Homoeopathy sits on a three legged stool. What this means is that if a remedy has at least three symptoms in the same strength as your patients symptoms then that remedy is a potential cure for their condition or if not cure it will offer relief. Go to the library and take out a book that easily explains Homoeopathy especially in the making of the potencies.

Homeopathy Dosage Directions

Select the remedy that most closely matches the symptoms. In conditions where self-treatment is appropriate, unless otherwise directed by a physician, a lower potency (6X, 6C, 12X, 12C, 30X, or 30C) should be used. In addition, instructions for use are usually printed on the label.

Many homeopathic physicians suggest that remedies be used as follows: Take one dose and wait for a response. If improvement is seen, continue to wait and let the remedy work. If improvement lags significantly or has clearly stopped, another dose may be taken. The frequency of dosage varies with the condition and the individual. Sometimes a dose may be required several times an hour; other times a dose may be indicated several times a day; and in some situations, one dose per day (or less) can be sufficient. If no response is seen within a reasonable amount of time, select a different remedy.

What to Do If It Is All Too Hard

Most of the time in my books you normally have a list under the disease of all the Homoeopathic remedies commonly used for them with a little write up on how they are different. If you are having difficulties especially in a chronic disease condition and are house bound most of the time, what I want you to do is go to a Professional Homoeopath or even better get them to visit you at home so they can see the patient in their natural conditions. What I would like you to get from this is a remedy that covers all of your conditions. While he is there I would also like you to get separate remedies for the other medical conditions or aggravations which you could use as and when needed as each condition flares up. I want to empower you and put you in control of your circumstances and lessen the burden. A Homoeopath that sees you at home gets a far better idea of your problems and how they affect your life and makes it easier for them to match you to the right remedy and also makes it easier for them to prescribe for other acute conditions that come around from the chronic one. Be aware that he will ask similar questions as I have already mentioned so have a good read of the questions list so you will know what to expect and are able to give them an accurate answer. Homoeopaths want to know your mind, sleeping patterns, what makes you feel better and what makes your condition worse; they are like detectives trying to piece together a picture of you in the present moment of time which is what we call a person picture. So think of these questions you will be asked.